T0327595

IMMUNOASSAYS

ESSENTIAL DATA SERIES

Series Editors

D. Rickwood
Department of Biology, University of Essex,
Wivenhoe Park, Colchester, UK

B.D. Hames
Department of Biochemistry and Molecular Biology,
University of Leeds, Leeds, UK

Published titles

Centrifugation
Gel Electrophoresis
Light Microscopy
Vectors
Human Cytogenetics
Animal Cells: culture and media
Cell and Molecular Biology
PCR
Nucleic Acid Hybridization
Immunoassays

Forthcoming titles

Transcription Factors
Enzymes in Molecular Biology
Neuropeptides

See final pages for full list of titles and order form

IMMUNOASSAYS
ESSENTIAL DATA

Edited by

R. Edwards

NETRIA, St Bartholomew's Hospital, London, UK

JOHN WILEY & SONS

Chichester · New York · Brisbane · Toronto · Singapore

Published in association with BIOS Scientific Publishers Limited

© 1996 John Wiley & Sons Ltd, Baffins Lane, Chichester, West Sussex PO19 1UD, UK, tel (01243) 779777. Published in association with BIOS Scientific Publishers Ltd, 9 Newtec Place, Magdalen Road, Oxford OX4 1RE, UK.

British Library Cataloguing in Publication Data
A catalogue record for this book is available from the British Library.

ISBN 0 471 95275 3

Library of Congress Cataloging in Publication Data
Immunoassays: essential data/edited by R. Edwards.
   p. cm.—(Essential data series)
   ISBN 0-471-95275-3 (alk. paper)
   1. Immunoassay.   I. Edwards, Ray.   II. Series.
QP519.9.I42I438 1996
616.07'56——dc20
                                                95-49525
                                                     CIP

Typeset by Marksbury Multimedia Ltd, Bath, UK
Printed and bound by CPI Antony Rowe, Eastbourne

CONTENTS

Contents

Contents

CONTRIBUTORS

S. Blincko
NETRIA, St Bartholomew's Hospital-Royal Hospitals NHS
Trust, London EC1A 7BE, UK

R. Edwards
NETRIA, St Bartholomew's Hospital-Royal Hospitals NHS
Trust, London EC1A 7BE, UK

I. Howes
NETRIA, St Bartholomew's Hospital-Royal Hospitals NHS
Trust, London EC1A 7BE, UK

J. Little
NETRIA, St Bartholomew's Hospital-Royal Hospitals NHS
Trust, London EC1A 7BE, UK

ABBREVIATIONS

Ab	antibody
ABEI	aminobutyl ethyl isoluminol
ABTS	2,2′-azino-di(3-ethylbenzothiazoline-6-sulfonate)
AFP	alphafetoprotein
Ag	antigen
ALTM	all laboratory trimmed means
AM	activity modulation
ANOVA	analysis of variance
AP	alkaline phosphatase
AS	antiserum
BG	β-galactosidase
BSA	bovine serum albumin
DEAE	diethylaminoethyl
DELFIA	dissociation-enhanced luminescence fluorimmunoassay
DID	double immunodiffusion
DMF	dimethyl formamide
EIA	enzyme-labeled immunoassay
ELISA	enzyme-labeled immunosorbent assay
IFMA	immunofluorometric assay
IH	immunohistochemistry
IMA	immunometric assay
IRMA	immunoradiometric assay
IRP	international reference preparations
K	equilibrium constant
KLH	keyhole limpet hemacyanin
LIA	luminoimmunoassay
mcAb	monoclonal antibody
MDH	malate dehydrogenase
NSB	nonspecific binding
PACIA	particle counting immunoassay
PBS	phosphate buffered saline
PC	particle counting
PCS	photon correlation spectroscopy
PEG	polyethylene glycol
PETINIA	particle enhanced turbimetric inhibition immunoassay
PFIA	polarization fluoroimmunoassay

EQAS	external quality assessment schemes
FCS	fetal calf serum
FIA	fluoroimmunoassay
FITC	fluorescein isothiocyanate
FPR	false positive rate
GA	gluteraldehyde
GCV	geometric coefficient of variation
GC–MS	gas chromatography–mass spectroscopy
GO	glucose oxidase
GPD	glucose-6-phosphate dehydrogenase
HAT	hypoxanthine aminopterin and thymidine
HRP	horseradish peroxidase
HSA	human serum albumin
HT	hypoxanthine and thymidine
IA	immunoassay
ICMA	immunochemiluminometric assay
ICRP	International Commission on Radiological Protection
IE	immunoelectrophoresis
IEMA	immunoenzymetric assay
PH	passive hemaglutination
PL	proximal linkage
PNP	p-nitrophenylphosphate
QC	quality control
RBC	red blood cells (erythrocytes)
RER	response error relationship
RIA	radiolabeled immunoassay
RID	radioimmunodiffusion
ROC	receiver operator characteristics
RPH	reverse passive hemaglutination
SATA	n-succinimidyl s-acetylthioacetate
SMCC	succinimidyl 4-(N-maleimido-methyl) cyclohexane-1-carboxylate
SRID	single radial immunodiffusion
TOPO	tri-n-octylphosphine oxide
TPR	true positive rate
USERIA	ultrasensitive enzymic radioimmunoassay
WB	western blot
WSC	water soluble carbodiimides

PREFACE

Although the development of immunoassays began at the end of the 19th century, their potential has only been fully appreciated during the last couple of decades. Immunoassays are used to measure more substances than any other analytical technique and are applied in all the major disciplines. They also seem to occur in an inexhaustible variety of formats.

Acronyms, e.g. **PRIST**s, **SOPHIA**s etc., are used extensively which, whilst making reference to individual methods simpler, often obscure the generic principles involved. The general picture has been rather confused. One of the aims of this data book is to give a comprehensive reference for all categories of immunoassays without losing essential details and to provide a useful basis for classification.

In general, data have been limited to the best of current methodology. However, in reviewing photoluminescent labels (fluorophores in particular) efforts have been made to include some new and interesting compounds as this is an expanding field.

The constraints of space have necessitated the briefest mention of some subjects but, as far as possible, an extensive list of references has been included. It has only been possible to include a limited reference to commercially available immunoreagents, kits and automated analysis. The reader should use the two directories listed under suppliers and refer directly to manufacturers.

R. Edwards

Chapter 1 HISTORY AND CLASSIFICATION – R. Edwards

1 Introduction

Immunoassays are the most widely used analytical techniques and have been successfully applied to an extensive range of substances, including both large and small molecules, cells, cellular components and viruses. They depend on the use of selected specific antibodies as reagents. Because antibodies can display high specificity and can react with high affinity, immunoassays are capable of measuring substances in complex matrices without pre-treatment, extraction, purification or concentration. This simplicity of application and the concomitant high throughput are essential aspects of immunoassays.

2 Historical development

The development of immunoassays has spanned the century.

Table 1 indicates some of the important stages in the early evolution of immunoassay procedures.

3 Classification and terminology

There is no consistent view on classification or terminology with respect to immunoassays. The fundamental principle is that an immunoassay is an analytical method that depends upon an antigen–antibody reaction and in a broad sense is usually quantitative. However, subsequent divisions can be made in a number of different ways and there is a plethora of variations possible, thus a coherent, universal scheme has never been adopted. A broad scheme useful for both classification and terminology preferred by the authors is outlined in *Figure 1*. A glossary of the terms used in immunoassay is given in *Table 2*.

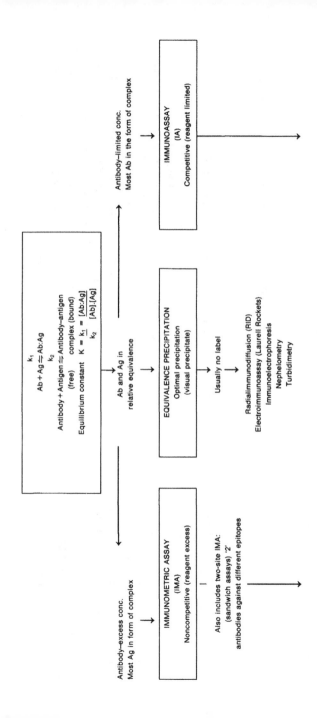

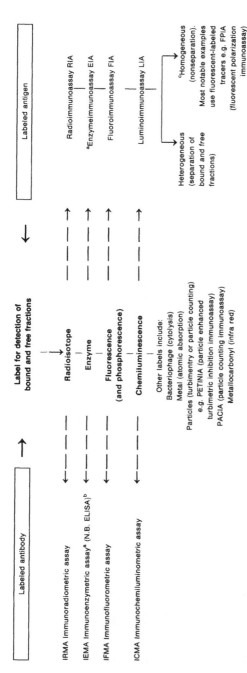

Figure 1. A classification system for immunoassays. [a]Choice of substrates yielding spectrum of detection signals, e.g. (i) radiolabeled substrate–ultrasensitive enzymic radioimmunoassay (USERIA); (ii) fluorescent product; (iii) enhanced chemiluminescent signal; (iv) cofactor cycling enzyme amplification. [b]ELISA (enzyme-labeled immunosorbent assay) is usually an immunometric assay where the labeled antibody is bound by solid-phase antigen. [c]Other homogeneous systems include enzyme-labeled tracers.

History and Classification

3

Table 1. Historical development of immunoassays

Date	Authors	Subject	Ref.
1890s	Krause	Reaction of soluble antigen and antiserum	1
1903	Uhlenhuth	Improved sensitivity of precipitin reaction	2
1905	Bechold	Analysis of individual antigen–antiserum reactions in complex mixtures by applying diffusion in gel techniques	3
1917	Landsteiner	'Artificial Conjugated Antigen', later to be described as hapten	4
1929	Heidelberger and Kendall	Quantitative immunochemical method using precipitin reaction	5
1941	Coons	Labeling antibody with fluorophore	6
1946	Oudin	Immunological analysis by tube diffusion method in agar gel using simple and double diffusion	7
1947	Ouchterlony	Formation of immune precipitate in gel plates using simple diffusion in two dimensions and double diffusion in one and two dimensions	8
1954	Stavitsky and Arquila	Quantitative immunoassay utilizing hemagglutination	9, 10
1960	Ekins; Berson and Yalow	Radioimmunoassay (RIA)	11, 12
1967	Wide; Miles and Hales	Radiolabeled antibody technique, i.e. immunoradiometric assay (IRMA)	13–15
1968	Haberman; Wide; Addison and Hales	Two-site IRMA. Use of two different antibodies to enhance specificity	
1976	Kohler and Milstein	Monoclonal antibody; production of antibodies with monospecificity and potentially inexhaustible supply *in vitro*	16

Table 2. Glossary of common terms in immunoassay

Term	Definition
Affinity	Strength of the association between antibody and antigen, a thermodynamic expression of the primary binding energy
Allotype	Site shared in common by groups of immunoglobulins. Anti-allotypic antibodies are those that recognize and bind to common epitopes (in the constant region) of antibodies (see Idiotype)
Analyte	That which is measured, often synonymous with the term antigen in immunoassays
Antigen	That which generated the antibody and specifically binds to the antibody binding site (see Analyte)
Avidity	Potential antigen binding capacity of antibody; related to affinity and number of binding sites
Biphasic response	See Hook
Bound (fraction)	Proportion of analyte (or labeled analyte) bound to antibody (see Free)
Coating	Process of passive absorption of antibodies by plastic surface, as in coated' tube
Complex	Usually refers to the antibody–antigen bound complex with multivalent binding
Conjugate	Often refers to an antigen or hapten covalently linked to a label, e.g. antigen–enzyme
Cross reactivity	Relative potency (as %) of substances other than antigen (but usually sharing some molecular similarity) with the antibody
Double antibody	See Second antibody
Epitope	That part of the antigen that reacts with the antibody binding site, i.e. antigenic determinant
Free (fraction)	Proportion of analyte (or labeled analyte) not bound to antibody (see Bound)
Free (hormone)	Refers to the measurement of that part of circulating hormone not bound by carrier' protein. N.B. not to be confused with 'Free fraction' (see above)
Hapten	A small molecular entity which will bind with an antibody binding site but requires coupling to a larger molecule to elicit an immune response (i.e. to generate an antibody response)

Continued

History and Classification

5

Table 2. Glossary of common terms in immunoassay, *continued*

Term	Definition
Heterogeneous	immunoassays requiring physical separation of bound and free fractions (*see* Homogeneous)
Heteroscedasticity	Nonuniformity of error in the response variable. This is a common feature of immunoassays
Homogeneous	Immunoassays where bound or free fractions are discriminated without separation (*see* Heterogeneous)
Hook	Dose–response relationship that inverts (i.e. 'hooks'), sometimes referred to as 'biphasic'. This phenomenon is seen in some immunometric assays (IMAs) and could give rise to misleading results
Idiotype	Unique site on individual immunoglobulin molecules. Anti-idiotypic antibodies are those that recognize and bind a part (in the hypervariable region) of a unique antibody. (e.g. bind to the hapten binding site (*see* Allotype'))
Label	Synonym for labeled antigen. The antigen or at least that molecular entity that binds to a specific binding site 'labeled' with a moiety to facilitate detection (e.g. radioisotope, enzyme, fluorophore, etc.)
Matrix	Medium used as a base for making standards (*see* Standards) or quality control pools (e.g. solution of various proteins, serum, etc.)
Misclassification error	The measurement of part of the bound fraction as free or vice versa
Non-specific binding (NSB)	The proportion of 'labeled' antigen (*see* Label) that is measured in the bound fraction but is not bound to the specific binding site
Second antibody	An antibody raised in a 'second' species against the immunoglobulins of the primary species (e.g. donkey anti-rabbit). Usually used to form a precipitable complex
Standard	Usually refers to the material used to calibrate the assay, hence 'standard' curve when referring to dose–response relationship
Titer	The dilution of an antiserum giving a specific response (e.g. 50% binding of labeled antigen)
Tracer	Synonym for 'labeled' antigen (*see* Label)
Zero binding	Binding of labeled antigen in the absence of analyte (unlabeled antigen), often referred to as B_0

Chapter 2 ANTIBODIES AND ANTISERA – R. Edwards

1 Antibodies

An important aspect of the immune response is the production of antibodies or immunoglobulins, an heterogeneous group of glycoproteins present in the serum and tissues, by B-cell lymphocytes. Serum, when it contains specified antibodies, is referred to as antiserum.

All antibodies have the same basic structure of four polypeptide chains: two identical 'light' chains and two identical 'heavy' chains, linked together by disulfide bonds in a distinctive Y conformation (*Figure 1*).

Immunoglobulins are divided into classes (IgG, IgM, IgE, IgA and IgD) and subclasses (e.g. IgG_1, IgG_2, etc).

IgG class immunoglobulins in animal sera constitute about 75% of total serum immunoglobulins (see *Table 1*).

Antibodies produced by hyperimmunization are predominantly IgG, occasionally with IgM. IgM antibodies are often less stable.

2 Production of antibodies

The initial stimulation of antibody production is usually achieved in an animal following the injection of an immunogen. Some antigens are immunogenic; that is, they will elicit an immune response which includes the production of antibodies when administered into an animal such as a rabbit. The key factors that confer immunogenicity are molecular size and defined tertiary structure. Generally, small molecules are less immunogenic than larger ones and it is likely that molecules smaller than about 3000 Da are not immunogenic. If an antigen is either not immunogenic or only weakly immunogenic, it should be coupled to an

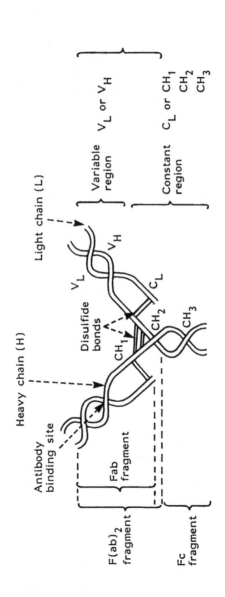

Figure 1. Diagram of an antibody molecule. $F(ab)_2$: from limited proteolytic digestion with full antigen binding activity. Fc: binds complement, binds to cellular Fc receptors, responsible for Fc–Fc interactions, important in Ab–Ag aggregates, interacts with phagocytic factors.

immunogenic carrier, as described in section 3, before administration.

Antisera may be raised successfully in several different animal species. Rabbit and sheep have been used extensively.

2.1 Production of polyclonal antisera

The administration of an immunogen *in vivo* will stimulate different cells of the immune system, giving rise to a mixed population of antibodies derived from a number of B-lymphocyte clones (polyclonal). Serum taken from an immunized animal containing these antibodies is referred to as a polyclonal antiserum.

The immunization of animals and subsequent handling is subject to regulations and legislation; as such it is best done by, or under the guidance of, an experienced expert. There are many commercial sources of polyclonal antisera and custom antiserum. (e.g. SAPU, PAL, Guildhay, TCS, Fitzgerald, Seralab, Scripps, Scantibodies and Sigma). A broad outline of an immunization schedule is given in [1].

2.2 Production of monoclonal antibodies [2]

Monoclonal antibody (mcAb) production has rapidly become established practice, although involving a variety of approaches. Kohler and Milstein's original method [3] was to fuse B-cell antibody producers with neoplastic tumor cells (B-cell myeloma), producing immortal hybrid cells or 'hybridomas'.

For reasons of history and convenience, most monoclonal work has been, and will continue, with the mouse. From a practical point of view, it is usually preferable to source mcAbs from the large number available commercially (e.g. BioChem ImmunoSystems, Biogenesis, Chemicon, Fitzgerald, Genzyme, SAPU, Scripps, Scantibodies and Seralab), or to consider custom production on a contract basis. The in-house' development of mcAb is an expensive undertaking requiring considerable investment of time, money and expertise with speculative results.

The conventional approach using immunized mice and mouse-derived myeloma cell lines consists of four aspects:

Antibodies and Antisera

1. immunization;
2. cell fusion;
3. cloning;
4. culturing and purification.

Purification of mcAb from either culture medium or ascitic fluid can be achieved using one of the techniques given in section 4 (below). The method chosen depends to a great extent on the degree of purity required.

3 Conjugated haptens

When an antigen is not immunogenic or only weakly immunogenic, it will be necessary to couple it to an immunogenic carrier in order to effect an antibody response. The main factor governing the potential immunogenicity is molecular size.

The following rule of thumb can be used to assess immunogenicity, and hence the need to couple to a carrier.

aldehyde to couple via amine groups; the mixed anhydride reaction to specifically activate carboxyl groups before reacting with amine groups; and the carbodiimide reaction to couple carboxyl groups and amine groups. These coupling reactions can lead to cross-linking of either antigen or carrier.

The molar ratio of coupled peptide to carrier is important for the production of good antisera. Satisfactory molar ratios are at least 10:1 for BSA; 20:1 for thyroglobulin; and 80:1 for KLH.

4. Purification of antibodies

Although antibodies are used as immunoreagents in their native form (e.g. in serum, ascitic fluid or culture medium), purification can confer benefits and in some cases is a prerequisite to satisfactory performance (see *Table 2*).

The IgG fraction of an antiserum contains antibodies of

1. Molecular weight < 3000 – probably not immunogenic, couple to carrier.
2. Molecular weight 3000–5000 – weakly immunogenic, coupling to carrier should enhance immunogenicity.
3. Molecular weight 5000–10 000 – probably immunogenic, coupling may enhance immunogenicity.
4. Molecular weight $> 10\ 000$ – should be immunogenic, usually no need to couple to carrier.

Various immunogenic carriers have been used, the most common being:

1. bovine serum albumin (BSA) or human serum albumin (HSA);
2. rabbit thyroglobulin;
3. keyhole limpet hemacyanin (KLH).

KLH and thyroglobulin are considered to be better carriers for small molecules and to give rise to antibodies with high affinity. However, BSA has been found to be satisfactory for many peptides. Three general methods are given: glutar-

hundreds of different specificities, derived from different B-cell clones and most of which are irrelevant for the purposes of immunoassay. It is often useful to make partially purified IgG protein from antisera, e.g. by salt precipitation, particularly when preparing solid phases.

In order to label polyclonal antibodies, more extensive purification is necessary (i.e. isolation of specific antibody by affinity chromatography using immobilized antigen). This procedure is obligatory because the presence of labeled irrelevant antibody, as well as labeled nonimmunoglobulin protein, adversely affects immunoassay performance.

The development of mcAb technology has greatly simplified the preparation of pure and specific immunoreagents, particularly labeled antibody. Highly purified, monospecific and well-characterized antibodies for many common analytes are now available commercially. The initial high purity and homogeneity means easy and reproducible labeling and simplified purification of the products.

5 Characterization and selection of antibodies or antisera

There are three factors necessary for judicious selection of antibodies or antisera:

1. concentration of binding sites;
2. affinity;
3. specificity.

It is therefore important to detail or indicate aspects of these in order to characterize all antibodies or antisera if they are to be used as immunoreagents. The most practical tests are:

1. determination of titer. This is a measure of both concentration and affinity;
2. Scatchard analysis of binding curve. This gives details of both affinity and number of binding sites;
3. cross-reaction studies with structurally related molecules. This can give information to describe the type and degree of specificity.

B, specifically bound labeled antigen after subtracting nonspecific binding;

F, calculated by subtracting *B* from Total activity determined in presence of excess antibody;

B/F, dividing *B* by *F* for each concentration;

[B], calculate concentration of specifically bound antigen from total for antigen + total for labeled antigen x %*B* (*B* as % of Total), for each concentration.

2. Plot *B/F* as *y* variable and [B] as *x* variable.
3. Fit straight line through data points. Calculate gradient to find **K** (equilibrium constant for the antibody–antigen reaction). The intercept on the *x* axis gives the total concentration of binding sites measurable under assay conditions. In a mixed population of antibodies Scatchard analysis may yield a curve which needs resolution into two or more straight lines.

5.3 Cross-reactions [4, 5]

Molecules structurally related to each antigen are used to determine the potential specificity of any given antiserum or antibody. Each cross-reactant will give a relative potency in

5.1 Determination of titer

The titer has been used extensively as a measure of quality. Although it does not necessarily denote quality, depending on both concentration and affinity of the antibodies, in practice antisera with high titers often exhibit high binding affinities. Satisfactory affinity of binding can be demonstrated using two antiserum dilution curves in the presence and absence of a minimum concentration of antigen. Displacement between the two curves denotes adequate sensitivity which in turn denotes an appropriate affinity.

5.2 Scatchard analysis [2]

Scatchard analysis of binding data is derived from a ratio of specifically bound antigen to free antigen (B/F) plotted against the concentration of specifically bound antigen ([B]). This plot is capable of giving an estimate of the binding affinity (i.e. K or equilibrium constant) and the number of available binding sites per unit volume.

Calculations for Scatchard analysis

1. Calculate the following for each concentration:

terms of binding compared with the specific antigen. Appropriate selection of cross-reactants differing in various parts of the molecule indicate the specificity of the antibody for particular parts of the molecule.

Table 1. Serum immunoglobulin concentrations

Class	Subclass	Human (mg ml^{-1})	Mouse (mg ml^{-1})
IgG		8–16	3–20
	IgG$_1$	5–10	6.5
	IgG$_{2a}$	1.8–3.0	4.2
	IgG$_{2b}$		1.2
	IgG$_3$	0.6–1.2	—
	IgG$_4$	0.3–0.6	—
IgM		0.5–2.0	0.1–1.0
IgA		1.4–4.0	1.0–3.0
IgD		0.0–0.4	0.0–0.01
IgE		10^{-4}–10^{-3}	10^{-4}–10^{-3}

Antibodies and Antisera

13

Table 2. Purification of antisera and antibodies

Method	Description	Ref.
IgG-enriched preparations		
Ammonium sulfate	40–45% saturated – mild method to precipitate IgG	6
Sodium sulfate	18% (w/v) – purer than ammonium sulfate but not as mild	6
Octanoic acid	Caprylic – leaves IgG in supernatant. Pure preparation	6
Ion-exchange purification of IgG		
DEAE ion exchange	Purify IgG-enriched fraction at pH 8.0 on column	6
Affinity chromatography of IgG		
Protein A	Strong affinity for Fc portion of IgG	e.g. Pharmacia
Protein G	Similar to Protein A	
Affinity purification of antibodies		
Immunosorbent	Elute specific antibodies with decreasing pH in presence of hydrophobic solvent e.g. 20% acetonitrile	7
Purified antibody fragments		
Fab, F(ab)₂ and Fc	Digestion of any of above fractions using pepsin or papain	8

Chapter 3 ASSAY DESIGN – R. Edwards

1 Introduction

The development of an immunoassay can be subdivided into four stages as follows:

1. selection of assay methodology;
2. selection of reagents;
3. optimization of assay conditions;
4. validation of assay protocol.

Although these are essentially consecutive steps, in practice some procedures run concurrently.

2 Selection of methodology

The selection of an appropriate methodology is governed by only a few simple principles but should also be guided by factors such as available expertise, equipment and cost. It is

clear that certain methods are more suitable for particular applications, and essentially the choice is based on aspects of the analyte.

2.1 Concentration of analyte

The target concentration of analyte (i.e. the concentration requiring maximum precision) determines to some extent the methodology used. *Figure 1* gives an indication of the relationship in broad terms. The immunometric assay (IMA) technique is potentially more sensitive than immunoassay (IA) techniques.

2.2 Molecular size of analyte

In general IAs are particularly suitable for small molecules and IMAs more suitable for large molecules. The equiva-

2.5 Other aspects

Cost can be a significant factor in choice of method. Because it only requires a simple spectrophotometer and simple reagents, the turbidimetric measurement of proteins is inexpensive. The use of radioisotopes as labels in immunoassays can often be restricted by legislation. Restrictions of patent legislation may constrain the use or availability of reagents in some technologies such as time-resolved fluorescence, enzyme amplification by co-factor cycling and enhanced chemiluminescence.

3 Selection of reagents

3.1 Selection of antibody

K value

The most important characteristic in selecting an antibody is the equilibrium (affinity) constant, the K value. For any given system, K will depend upon the particular antibody.

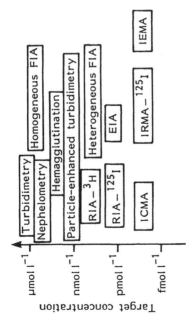

Figure 1. Diagram to show relationship between 'target concentration' and methodology. These positions depend on so many factors that they can only be given approximately.

lence precipitation methods, (e.g. gel diffusion) are most suited to larger molecules with a number of epitopes for rapid formation of multivalent precipitation complexes.

2.3 Expected range of analyte concentration

IAs seldom have a useful working range much beyond 10–100-fold. The range can obviously be extended artificially by concentration or dilution of the sample. If suitably developed, IMAs can have extended working ranges of several 1000-fold. A solid-phase antibody can be used to concentrate the analyte by an immunosorbent step, for more sensitive assays.

2.4 Specificity

The main constraint of specificity is in the choice of antibody (see Section 3.1 in this chapter); however, the choice of method can be pertinent. High background measurements by some techniques (e.g. simple fluorescence with complex biological specimens) can restrict specificity particularly in homogeneous (nonseparation) formats.

The 'two-site' IMA with antibodies directed towards different epitopes can be used to improve specificity,

This can be calculated using the Scatchard plot (see Chapter 2).

Antibodies associated with high K values are used to develop assays with greater sensitivity and vice versa. *Figure 2* can be used as a guide for selecting appropriate values.

Specificity

Antibodies should also be selected on the basis of specificity. Calculation of cross reactions (see Chapter 2) by relative potency gives a useful indication. It is for the assay developer to predict the degree of specificity required with respect to various epitopes. Specificity of polyclonal antisera can be enhanced by affinity purification (see Chapter 2).

Type

Monoclonal antibodies theoretically display monospecificity (i.e. react with a single epitope). Polyclonal antisera often contain antibodies which react with a number of different epitopes, but nonetheless display excellent specificity. In some assays it is necessary to respond to various epitopes,

Assay Design

Immunoassays

3.3 Selection of suitable matrix

A matrix is required for both standards (calibrants) and control samples. A suitable matrix is one without any analyte and which mimics the behavior of the sample matrix in the assay. If the exact composition of the sample matrix is known and is reasonably simple then an analyte-free matrix can be synthesized. Complex matrices, like serum, can be stripped of endogenous analyte using techniques like resin or charcoal adsorption or solid phase immunoaffinity extraction. Where there is immunodistinction of analyte between different species, matrix (e.g. serum) from one species can be used in assays for another (e.g. horse serum in assays for human analyte).

3.4 Selection of standard

One simple rule is that the standard material should be pure. It should also be identical to the analyte in the specimen. Both the quantity (available stocks) and stability should be such as permits reasonable continuity.

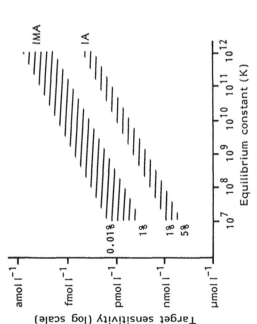

Figure 2. Relationship between target sensitivity and K value. Percentage figures indicate nonspecific binding (NSB) values.

The standard can be calibrated against reference materials such as international reference preparations (IRP) or material of chemical purity with defined mass.

3.5 Selection of separation reagents
See Chapter 4.

3.6 Selection of labeled tracer
See Chapters 5–7.

4. Optimization of assay conditions

There is a diversity of techniques and formats, thus it is only feasible to give a general outline of the principles involved. There has been considerable debate on the optimal strategy of assay development and in particular the advantages of either theoretical optimization or an empirical approach. In fact, most immunoassays have their uses. To develop most immunoassays some empirical steps are necessary as it is not possible to

particularly those used for screening procedures. A mixture of monoclonal antibodies can substitute for polyclonal antisera. Once the required monoclonal antibody is produced, supply can be maintained indefinitely. In general, polyclonal antisera are very stable and can be stored for several years with no loss of performance. Monoclonal antibodies are sometimes less stable and do not always precipitate satisfactorily in conventional techniques. Hence solid-phase systems are usually preferred.

3.2 Selection of buffer and components
Simple buffers with a physiological pH are used extensively as a medium in many immunoassay methods, for example:

0.05 M phosphate buffer, pH 7.4;
0.02 M Tris buffer, pH 7.4;
0.01 M Hepes buffer, pH 7.4;
mostly containing 0.15M sodium chloride.

The increase in molarity is thought to reduce nonspecific reactions. A number of different additives are used for a variety of purposes (*Table 1*).

Assay Design

19

identify and characterize all the theoretical factors and relationships. On the other hand, the use of theoretical studies has undoubtedly clarified several broad principles in contradiction of wrongly held beliefs.

The authors have found the theoretical studies and formulations of Ekins and co-workers [1–3] to be particularly useful in providing a framework for design and the general direction of subsequent empirical steps.

A suitable outline of assay development can be summarized as follows:

1. relative concentrations of reagents;
2. temperature of reaction;
3. reaction time;
4. reduction of errors.

All assay development (where the application is fully quantitative) should be assessed by reference to precision profiles [4] (see Chapter 11) and not by comparison of dose–response curves.

position is to use an amount of antibody to give a 10- to 20-fold increase in maximum specific binding over the NSB (i.e. 20% specific binding for 1% NSB) in an IA and 100- to 200-fold increase for an IMA.

The concentration of tracer is often governed by more functional aspects such as the need to limit the concentration to reduce the risk of contamination with radioactive tracers or not to exceed an optical density (OD) of 3–4 for an enzyme-labeled tracer. Too little radioactivity would increase the counting error for a given counting time (see Chapter 5).

The volume of sample is often adjusted to correspond to the sensitivity of the assay (i.e. more sample to compensate for insufficient sensitivity or vice versa). For samples with complex matrices (e.g. serum) it is inadvisable to exceed 20% of total volume.

4.2 Temperature of reaction

There are generally only a few variants of reaction temperature:

4.1 Relative concentrations of reagents

The optimal concentration of reagents depends upon a complexity of factors, in particular:

1. equilibrium constant (K);
2. sensitivity required;
3. specific activity of labeled analyte (tracer);
4. experimental error;
5. misclassification error; error in measurement of ratio of 'bound' to 'free'.

Given an antibody with appropriate constant and a requirement for optimal sensitivity, the concentration of antibody (in terms of univalent binding site) can be selected as 3/K and tracer as 4/K in an IA and more (possibly 10 times) for an IMA.

For more sensitivity (i.e. greater precision at very low concentrations) use less antibody. For less sensitivity but greater precision at higher concentrations, use more antibody.

The optimal concentration of antibody is intimately linked to the nonspecific binding (NSB) value. A useful starting

1. 4°C can minimize interfering reactions, e.g. in second antibody reaction;
2. Ambient (approx. 20°C–30°C) is often adequate;
3. 37°C increases rate and is physiological.

Although antibodies are very stable, even at elevated temperatures, other components could be susceptible to degradation or instability.

4.3 Reaction time

In order to shorten assay time it is necessary to increase temperature (see above) and/or concentration of reagents. An increase in concentration of reactants could compromise specificity. (In general as concentration increases specificity potentially decreases.)

4.4 Reduction of errors

The single most important contribution to improving or optimizing any immunoassay is by the reduction of NSB. This is effectively achieved by:

Assay Design

1. increasing molarity, e.g. by adding 0.15 M saline;
2. blocking surfaces by precoating with protein solutions, e.g. 1% BSA (w/v);
3. use of detergents, e.g. 0.5% (v/v) Tween 20, 0.1% (v/v) Triton X-100 and Triton X-405;
4. washing of antibody-bound fraction. This is usually much more effective if the antibody is adsorbed or coupled to a solid-phase surface. It is not usually necessary to exceed three washes. Two washes can often be adequate.

5 Validation

A developed assay protocol requires validation to establish suitability before proceeding to practical application. In broad terms validation should test the assay in the following ways:

1. recovery and dilution tests;
2. inter-assay precision;
3. response to interference;
4. comparison with reference method;
5. correlation with categories of specimen.

5.2 Inter-assay precision and drift

Assesses average precision profile for a number of assays including as many variables as would be relevant, e.g. different operators, different batches of reagents, etc. This should also indicate the mean sensitivity.

Drift is assessed in assays with a maximum number of specimens. Either quality control pools or various samples are repeatedly analyzed throughout the assay. A significant difference consistently raised or lowered throughout the assay would indicate a problem with drift.

5.3 Response to interference

Inappropriate responses to interfering factors or cross-reactants are difficult to assess in the absence of a totally reliable reference method. Measurements can be monitored for a change after the addition of suspected interfering factors or known cross-reactants.

Aspects of these tests can certainly be incorporated into the progressive development of an assay as outlined in the previous section. Nonetheless, they should be re-checked in the final format.

5.1 Recovery and dilution tests

Both these tests check that calibration is accurate and that the matrix is appropriate, but neither discriminates between the two.

Recovery

Measure the concentration in specimens before and after adding a known amount of pure analyte. The difference between the two measurements is expressed as a percentage of the added mass (i.e. optimal is 100% recovery).

Dilution

Measure concentration of specimens at various dilutions in matrix and assess linearity. Poor recovery or nonlinearity indicates inaccurate calibration or an inappropriate matrix or both.

It is sometimes possible to use regression analysis for groups of specimens that appear to be similar in all respects other than the presence or absence of interfering factors.

Typical interfering factors vary, depending on methods and applications. Some examples of interference are listed below:

1. sample specific effects, e.g. degradation due to hemoglobin, presence of lipids, etc;
2. effects of storage, e.g. time and temperature;
3. heterophilic antibodies;
4. rheumatoid factors;
5. antibodies reacting with label, e.g. anti-peroxidases or specific anti-mouse antibodies (present after patient treated with mouse monoclonal antibodies);
6. abnormal proteins, especially binding proteins;
7. high salt concentrations, e.g. urine;
8. chaotropic components, e.g. urea.

Immunoassays

5.4 Comparison with reference method

Results from the test protocol are compared with results on the same specimens obtained using a known reference' method. A suitable reference method is often one using definitive analytical steps, e.g. physico-chemical methods coupling chromatographic purification with specific detection such as gas chromatography–mass spectroscopy (GC–MS). Results are analyzed by linear regression analysis.

A useful reference target can also be provided by all laboratory trimmed means (ALTM) or method means for pooled source material distributed in external quality assessment schemes (EQAS).

5.5 Correlation with specified categories of specimens

The validity of this test is based on the assumption that mean results from groups of specimens would significantly differ in ways that would reflect respective categories, such as different pathologies.

Table 1. Buffer additives

Additive	Example	Reason
Protein	Bovine serum albumin 0.1–0.5% (w/v); gelatin 0.1–0.2% (w/v); serum 1–5% (v/v)	Reduce nonspecific binding of labeled tracer to various surfaces
Detergent	Triton X-100 0.01–0.1% (v/v); Tween 20 0.05–0.5% (v/v)	Reduce nonspecific binding to solid-phase reagents
Protease inhibitors	Trasylol (aprotinin); Bacitaracin	Eliminate degradation of certain components, especially the tracer, sensitive to protelytic activity usually originating with the specimen
Specific blocking agents	Salicilate; ANS (8-anilino-l-naphthalene sulfonic acid)	Eliminate binding of either analyte or labeled analyte to specific binding proteins
Specific proteins or serum	Gamma globulins; mouse serum	Remove effect of heterophilic antibodies or specific antiglobulin antibodies
Preservatives	Sodium azide 0.05–0.1% (w/v); Thiomersal 0.02% (w/v); Bronidox 0.1% (v/v)	Useful to prolong shelf life of buffers and prevent growth of micro-organisms
Others	EDTA 0.01 M: heparin (10 IU/tube)	Optimize second antibody reaction (see Chapter 4)
	PEG (polyethylene glycol 6000) 1.4% (w/v)	Enhances visual precipitation especially in turbidimetry

Assay Design

Chapter 4 SEPARATION – R. Edwards

1 Introduction

For all types of immunoassay, IAs and IMAs, some method of discriminating between 'bound' and 'free' moieties must precede measurement. It is necessary to discern the difference between bound and free analyte in IAs or bound and free antibody in IMAs.

Discrimination involves either:

1. a physical separation of bound and free fractions (i.e. heterogenous systems); or
2. a characteristic change in signal associated with antibody binding (i.e. homogeneous systems) (nonseparation).

2 Homogeneous systems

The error or nonspecific measurement in homogeneous

1. should not disturb equilibrium;
2. separation of bound and free should be complete;
3. have negligible or low NSB;
4. have negligible sample matrix interactions;
5. be quick and inexpensive.

Many different methods have been used with satisfactory results. However, there has been a definite trend towards more specific methods such as second antibody precipitation or a solid-phase reagent. The most significant factor has been a growing awareness of the need for low NSB. Specific methods invariably have low NSBs. Solid-phase reagents are easily washed to reduce the NSB considerably. The use of nonspecific separation methods is usually more practical where samples do not have complex matrices. Nonspecific separation methods are given in *Table 2* and specific types in

assays is high. This is because any change in signal following antibody binding is usually a matter of degree (i.e. partial) and not complete. The change may also be subject to interference. These constraints effect sensitivity and it is usual to find that homogeneous IAs or IMAs are applied to high concentrations of analyte. Examples of the major types of homogeneous systems are listed in *Table 1*.

3 Separation heterogeneous systems

The use of a separation step (i.e. heterogeneous system) gives more specificity, better precision and allows for measurement of much lower concentrations. The essential aspects of an ideal separation method are as follows:

Table 3. A few techniques that fit into neither category are listed in *Table 4*.

4 Chemistries for covalent coupling to solid-phase

Many solid-phases have specific reactive groups which can be activated by a variety of chemistries (see *Table 5*). Two-step procedures (i.e. activation followed by coupling) are considered to be more effective. One-step methods (i.e. with simultaneous activation and coupling may lead to polymerization of reagents and subsequent loss of immunoreactivity to solid-phases.

Separation

27

Table 1. Homogeneous systems

Change in signal			Ref.
Change in enzyme activity	(i)	Inhibition of enzyme activity due to steric restriction of active site following binding. Site of coupling to enzyme critical; difficult to predict	1
	(ii)	Activation of activity	2
Change in fluorescence	(i)	Quenching of polarized fluorescence due to faster rotational speed of unbound fluorescent labeled analyte	3
	(ii)	Quenching of fluorescence due to binding of antibody to fluorescent tracer	4
	(iii)	Enhancement of fluorescence due to antibody binding reduces impairment of fluorescent tracer	5
	(iv)	Indirect quenching of fluorophore by antifluorophore antibody is prevented by steric hindrance of anti-analyte antibody binding	6
	(v)	Quenching of fluorescence of one fluorophore by transfer of energy to second fluorophore in juxtaposition, brought about when antibody labeled with one fluorophore reacts with an analyte labeled with the other	7
Change in signal from radioisotope		The scintillation proximity assay principle relies on the generation of photons from scintillants incorporated in solid phase coupled to antibody when activated by bound radiolabeled analyte. Applicable with low energy radioisotope, i.e. ³H where unbound tracer does not activate scintillant	
		Three types:	
	(a)	fluorophore impregnated microparticles, e.g. SPA from Amersham;	8
	(b)	scintillant impregnated microtiter plates, e.g. ScintiStrips from Wallac;	
	(c)	scintillant layered on to bottom of microtiter wells, e.g. FlashPlates from DuPont-NEN	
Visual precipitate		Antibody and antigen in equivalent amounts react to produce a multivalent complex which gives rise to a visual precipitation line. The basis of many immunodiffusion plate techniques	9
Agglutination		Either antigen or antibody is coupled to particles, e.g. latex particles or red blood cells. Agglutination of the particles detected by eye as a measure of the analyte (either antibody or antigen)	10

Light scattering — Reaction of antibody and antigen in equivalent amounts producing insoluble molecular complexes which deflect light beam as in turbidimetry or nephelometry — 11

Table 2. Nonspecific separation methods

Method	Characteristics	Ref.
Electrophoretic (high voltage)	Original method used in first published RIA. Required high specific activity radioisotope, e.g. ^{131}I. Only method to detect degraded tracer and to correct for degree of degradation	12, 13
Gel exclusion chromatography	Has been used in automated system. Some potential but not commonly practical	14
Adsorption	(i) Dextran-coated charcoal used as a suspension to precipitate 'free'. Invariably requires refrigerated conditions especially for centrifugation. Usually rapid precipitation (provided fines are removed). Inexpensive, otherwise no longer recommended. Batch to batch variation. Not suitable for use with complex biological fluids such as serum	15
	(ii) Suspension of various silicates, e.g. Fullers earth, florisil, to precipitate 'free'. No longer recommended	16
	(iii) Adsorption of antibody (bound fraction) by hydroxyapatite	17
Fractional precipitation of proteins[a]	(i) Ethanol	18
	(ii) Ammonium sulphate approximately 1.8 M	18
	(iii) PEG (12–20% w/v PEG 6000)	18

[a] All these use well-defined products with little or no batch to batch variation. Inexpensive methods with limited application to either noncritical assays or with nonbiological samples.

29

Separation

Table 3. Specific separation methods

Method	Characteristics	Ref.
Second antibody (Ab_2)	Formation of precipitable complex using the reaction of antiserum raised against the specific animal immunoglobulins of the primary antibody (Ab_1), e.g. donkey anti-rabbit serum interacts with a rabbit antibody. May require carrier serum, ie. normal (nonimmune) serum, if AB_1 at low concentration, e.g. <1:10 000 dilution, e.g. Add 50 ml of 1:100 to 1:500 dilution of carrier serum (e.g. normal rabbit serum or normal sheep serum)	19, 20
	(i) Post-precipitation Precipitation reagents, i.e. Ab_2 and carrier serum added at end of primary reaction. Usually reacts for 24 h at 4°C Precipitation usually requires centrifugation >1000 *g* for >30 min at 4°C	
	(ii) Pre-precipitation Ab_1 and Ab_2 (also carrier serum if required) reacted together prior to use in immunoassay. Possible to use less Ab_2 because of extended reaction time. Can reduce interference of cross reacting immunoglobulins (e.g. in the sample) with Ab_2. Has not proved popular as it often restricts or interferes with the immunoreactivity of the primary reaction	
Assisted second antibody	(i) Dextran/Ab_2 Addition of dextran (e.g. 3% of Dextran 40) enhances precipitation	18
	(ii) Ammonium sulfate/Ab_2 Addition of ammonium sulfate (e.g. 1–1.2 M) enhances Ab_2 reaction	18
	(iii) PEG/Ab_2 Addition of polyethylene glycol (PEG) 6000 e.g. 4% solution, enhances Ab_2 reaction	21
Solid phase	One reagent, e.g. Ab_1 or Ab_2 coupled to solid phase material renders it insoluble and easily removed from reaction	

(i) Plastic surface — 22

Passive absorption of reagent onto plastic surface, e.g. polystyrene bead, tube or microtiter plate, by low molarity carbonate buffer pH 9.6

(ii) Modified plastic — 23

Covalent coupling to chemically modified plastic with surface reactive groups

(a) COOH groups

(b) NH$_2$ groups

e.g. microtiter plates for (a) and (b) from Costar and Nunc

(iii) Particles

(a) Agarose particles, e.g. microfine cellulose; covalent coupling to OH groups — 24

(b) Nylon fine suspension; covalent coupling to -NH$_2$ group — 25

(iv) Silanized particles — 26

Glass beads or particles silanized with silane derivatives containing reactive groups for covalent coupling

(v) Magnetizable particles — 27

(a) Cellulose based, e.g. from Sci-Pac — 24

(b) Polyacrolein based — 28

(c) Silanized ferric oxide — 28

(d) Core and shell particles, e.g. Dynospheres from Dyno — 29

(vi) Latex particles — 23

Microfine particles <0.1 µm up to 100 mm size, usually polystyrene also with chemically modified surface groups,

e.g. -COOH group

-CONH$_2$ groups

-NH$_2$ group

e.g. above available from Seradyn and Polymer Laboratories

Separation

31

Table 4. Other methods of separation

Method	Characteristics	Ref.
Polymerization	Cross-linking of antibodies by polymerization using glutaraldehyde or ethylchloroformate. More effective using filtration rather than centrifugation. Partial loss of immunoreactivity likely following polymerization	30
Entrapping	Entrapment of antibodies within interstitial spaces of water insoluble polymer, (e.g. polyacrylamide). The size of lattice may restrict access by larger molecules	31
Microencapsulation	Encapsulation of antibodies within a semi-permeable membrane, by forming a polymer (e.g. nylon, polyurea or cellulose nitrate) at interface of an emulsion. Used for measurement of small molecules	32
Biotin–avidin	Usually couple avidin (or streptavidin) to solid-phase and biotinylate reagent. The very high affinity of biotin for avidin will couple reagent to solid-phase during assay	33

Table 5. Solid-phase reactive groups

Solid-phase reactive group	Method	Ref.
Carboxylate	(i) Couple with water soluble carbodiimides (WSC) (ii) Convert to active ester by coupling N-hydroxysuccinimide using WSC (iii) Convert to NH₂ group by reacting with diamino alkane (introduces spacer arm)	28
Amide	React with hydrazine to produce hydrazide group then couple using difunctional groups, e.g. glutaraldehyde	28
Amine	Convert to carboxylate with spacer, e.g. succinic anhydride Couple with WSC or glutaraldehyde	28
Hydroxyl	Activation by: cyanogen bromide, tosyl chloride (p-toluene sulfonyl chloride), 2,2,2-trifluoroethane sulfonyl chloride, carbonyl-di-imidazole; then couple to -NH₂ groups	34, 35, 36, 37

N.B. Coupling procedures are usually more effective if they use two-step chemistries.

Chapter 5 RADIOLABELED IMMUNOASSAYS – R. Edwards

1 Introduction

Radioisotopes were first used as labeled tracers in immunoassays in the late 1950s, leading to important publications from two groups pivotal in the generation of radioimmunoassays (see Chapter 1). Although other labeled immunoassays had been published earlier, the use of a radioisotope conferred critical advantages (*Table 1*).

2 Radioisotopes used in immunoassays

A number of radioisotopes have been used as tracers in various immunoassays including ^{131}I, ^{75}Se and ^{14}C. At present there are only two commonly encountered radioisotopes, i.e. ^{125}I and ^{3}H. Characteristics of these are shown in *Table 2*. Occasionally ^{57}Co is used in dual label assays together with ^{125}I [1].

3 Radioactivity

Radioactivity is the emission of subatomic particles and radiation from unstable atomic nuclei when disintegrating spontaneously. See *Table 3* for a glossary of terms related to radioactivity.

3.1 Units for radioactivity
SI unit

The Becquerel (Bq) = one nuclear transformation (disintegration) per second (dps).

$1 \text{ Bq} = 1 \text{ dps} = 2.7 \times 10^{-11} \text{ Curie (Ci)}$

$1 \text{ Ci} = 3.7 \times 10^{10} \text{ Bq}$

Radiolabeled Immunoassays

3.2 Half-life ($t_{1/2}$)

The half-life ($t_{1/2}$) is the time taken for the number of parent nuclei to fall to half the number present at zero time (t_0) (i.e. the time taken for half the number of radioactive nuclei to disintegrate). Each radioisotope has a characteristic $t_{1/2}$.

4 Production of radiolabeled tracers

4.1 Tritiated tracers (^{3}H)

Most laboratories are not equipped to produce their own tritiated tracers. Many tritiated tracers with sufficiently high specific activities (i.e. >50 Ci mmol^{-1}, i.e. 1.85×10^{12} Bq mmol^{-1}) are routinely available from commercial suppliers, e.g. Amersham, DuPont NEN, CIS and ICN.

They are generally made by direct chemical synthesis such as:

1. catalytic reduction of unsaturated precursors with tritium gas;

4.3 Conjugation radiolabeling

The covalent coupling of a chemically reactive group containing a radioisotope to the tracer molecule is called conjugation radiolabeling. As an indirect labeling technique it is used where one of the direct labeling methods has proved ineffective or undesirable, usually for one of the following reasons:

1. direct labeling technique damages the tracer molecule, often through susceptibility to oxidation;

2. direct incorporation of radioisotope comprises the binding of an epitope to the binding site. This applies particularly to large molecules like radioiodine, but should not be relevant to incorporation of ^{3}H;

3. direct labeling not possible as tracer molecule does not contain appropriate moieties, e.g. radioiodination of peptide not possible through lack of group like tyrosine.

Generally, conjugation radiolabeling gives products with lower specific activity than those derived by direct labeling.

2. dehalogenation using tritium gas;
3. reduction of intermediate compounds with tritiated borohydride or radioisotope exchange reactions;
4. exchange of tritium for hydrogen, using tritium gas or tritiated water.

4.2 Radioiodinated tracers (^{125}I)

Radioiodine is readily incorporated into many molecules. It is supplied as high specific activity sodium ^{125}I-iodide (carrier free) from commercial sources, e.g. Amersham, NEN and CIS. The iodide is oxidized by one of the following methods to the reactive species, cationic iodine (*Table 4*). Radioiodination using lactoperoxidase is considered to be a mild process, reducing the possibility of damaging the tracer molecule. Both the chloramine T and the iodogen method have been used successfully for a variety of antigens. These protocols have been optimized to yield a product just less than 1 atom of radioiodine per molecule of tracer.

Where the conjugated product is readily purified from the reactants, such as with most hapten molecules (small molecules), the yield can be optimized by an excess of the antigenic reactant. ^{125}I-Bolton and Hunter reagent [3] *N*-succinimidyl 3-(4-hydroxy, 5-[^{125}I]iodophenyl) propionate is available commercially, e.g. Amersham, DuPont-NEN, at specific activity ~2000 Ci mmol^{-1} (~74 TBq mmol^{-1}). *N*-succinimidyl [2,3-^{3}H] propionate may be used to label with tritium in a similar manner.

5 Purification of radiolabeled tracers

The purity of the radiolabeled tracer is one of the most critical aspects of an immunoassay. High purity is essential for an optimal performance. Impure tracers will seriously compromise results. The choice of purification will be dictated by the following points:

1. molecular characteristics of product and reactants;
2. need to contain radioactivity, avoiding radiation hazards or potential contamination;

Radiolabeled Immunoassays

3. disposal of waste radioactivity.

Purification of the extensive range of molecules used in immunoassays requires a multitude of methods. *Table 5* gives selected examples together with salient features.

6 Assessment of radiolabeled tracer

A radiolabeled tracer can be assessed by its purity, specific activity and stability.

6.1 Purity

An indication of purity is made by a suitable chromatographic or electrophoretic profile of radioactivity. The highest level of purity is important for the successful application of immunoassay principles. This measure is not totally reliable due to absorption and loss of very small amounts of impurities during the separation, giving a falsely elevated value for purity.

material. This method assumes no difference of immunoreactivity in comparison with the unlabeled analyte.

6.3 Stability

Stability is measured empirically over an appropriate time interval. To enhance stability the radiolabeled tracer is stored at reduced temperature, diluted (by less than 700 kBq ml^{-1}) and in the presence of appropriate stabilizers (e.g. cysteine).

7 Detection

See *Table 6* for a glossary of terms related to counting.

7.1 Detection of ³H (Beta counters)

³H-tracers are measured using liquid scintillation counting. The energy of charged β-particles excites a chemical scintillant, which then emits photons of light. This light is quantified using photomultiplier tubes in a liquid scintilla-

Having established an acceptable radiolabeled tracer, the NSB value is often the single most effective monitor of variations in purity. An increase in NSB value (i.e. as percentage of total counts) indicates a concomitant decrease in purity.

6.2 Specific activity

Specific activity (radioactivity) = radioactivity per unit mass of an element or compound containing the radionuclide, e.g. $mCi\ mg^{-1}$, $kBq\ mg^{-1}$, $\mu Ci\ mmol^{-1}$, $MBq\ mmol^{-1}$, etc.

A simple estimate of specific activity can be calculated from the following equation:

Specific activity $(kBq\ \mu g^{-1}$ or $\mu Ci\ \mu g^{-1}) = $ (% incorporation of radioiodine (i.e. yield) x total radioactivity (kBq))/ mass of antigen (μg)

assuming no losses, and correcting for decay constant.

Where the mass of antigen is unknown, it is possible to generate a calibration curve using increasing amounts of radiolabeled

tion counter. Because the energy is low, sample and scintillant need to be in close proximity to ensure efficient energy transfer. The tracer is usually solubilized in a solution containing the appropriate scintillants.

Automated liquid scintillation counters with single or multiple detectors for use with vials, tubes, microtiter plates, flat filters and membranes are available from suppliers such as Wallac, Packard and ICN.

Nonseparation (homogeneous) using ³H-tracers

Homogeneous radiolabeled immunoassays (i.e. without a separation of bound and free) is possible if the scintillant is localized, e.g. in a bead or at a surface of a well. Commercial products are available from Amersham (SPA, Scintillation Proximity Assay), Wallac (ScintiStrip) and DuPont NEM (Flashplate).

7.2 Detection of ^{125}I (gamma counters)

Gamma radiation can be efficiently measured using a

Radiolabeled Immunoassays

thallium activated sodium iodide crystal (NaI) optically coupled to a photomultiplier.

Various manual or automated gamma counters with single well or multiple detectors are available from suppliers, e.g. Wallac, Packard and ICN.

7.3 Counting error

Radioactive decay is a random event and it is not possible to predict when any given atom will disintegrate. The counting error is a function of the probability of an unstable nucleus disintegrating or decaying.

Counting error $= \sqrt{\text{no of counts}}$

8 Regulation and legislation

8.1 Publications

The handling and use of radioisotopes is regulated and controlled by a number of publications. The intention of

8.2 Dose

A dose received is a function of the specific radioisotope and the type and energy of its radiation, the distance over which the radiation travels and the medium through which it travels (see *Table 7* for units of radiation dose).

8.21 Dose limits

Dose limits recommended by the ICRP were set at levels where there are negligible harmful effects. As distance increases, dose diminishes considerably (inverse square law). It is possible to estimate the average dose for a 'radioimmunoassayist' (e.g. a background dose of 10 μCi ^{125}I (unshielded), equivalent to a large assay batch, at a distance of 1 metre is 0.15 μSv h^{-1}. **It is clear that radiolabeled immunoassays do not present any hazard from direct radiation.**

Examples of typical doses to illustrate significance of dose limits are:

1. average annual dose for inhabitant of UK, 2.5 mSv;

these is to make users aware of certain recommended dose limits, to ensure that the doses of ionizing radiation received by classified persons are assessed in order to comply with the limits and to ensure that users demonstrate such compliance. They also control the disposal of radioactive waste.

Regulations controlling use of radioisotopes

1. *Recommendations of the International Commission on Radiological Protection (ICRP)*.
2. *Euratom Directive; Basic safety standards for radiation protection in the European Community*.
3. *The Health and Safety at Work Act, 1974, UK*.
4. *The Radioactive Substances Act, 1993, UK*.
5. *The Ionising Radiations Regulations, 1985, HMSO, UK*.
6. *Approved Code of Practice, 1985. The protection of persons against ionising radiations arising from any work activity. HMSO, UK*.
7. *The Federal Code of Regulations; together with Reports from the National Council for Radiation Protection (NCRP), USA*.

2. dose from single transatlantic flight, 0.04 mSv;
3. dose from an X-ray examination, up to 10 mSv;
4. average annual dose for radioimmunoassays using ^{125}I-tracers, approx. 0.03 mSv.

Unsealed radioactive sources used in radiolabeled immunoassays may irradiate body organs or tissues if ingested, inhaled or from surface contamination of the skin. The annual limit on intake, or the amount of radioisotope taken internally which produces the annual dose limit, varies for different isotopes (*Table 8*).

8.3 Specific applications to laboratory practice

Two basic areas of work are designated and are referred to as 'supervised areas' and 'controlled areas'. These areas are categorized by the amount of radioactivity present or the maximum dose (*Table 9*). Both categories are similar and would apply to the production of tracers, e.g. radioiodination procedures. They would not apply to analytical procedures.

Radiolabeled Immunoassays

Most laboratories using radiolabeled immunoassays would be designated as supervised areas on the basis of the derived limits of intake or surface contamination. It is a useful practice as it leads to better control, particularly of contamination and subsequent detrimental effects on detection and precision.

The design of a laboratory should allow easy supervision and monitoring of access. Proper laboratory design would involve a consultative process with the 'Radiation Protection Adviser'. Local rules would require additional constraints on high activity areas such as radioiodination suites.

Table 1. Critical advantages associated with the use of radioisotopes

Sensitivity	Potential sensitivities of 10^{-14} M depending on specific radioisotope
Specificity	Negligible background radiation in most samples and radioactivity not affected by analytical reactions or analytical environment, e.g. pH, molarity, etc.
Convenience	The use of radioiodine allowed for adaptable production of a wide range of tracers using simple laboratory procedures
Robust performance	Precise and efficient detection of radioactivity coupled with constancy of radioactivity
Low cost	Immunoassays using ^{125}I-tracers exemplify inexpensive analytical technique and low-cost detection

Table 2. Characteristics of principal radioisotopes used in immunoassays

Property	^{3}H	^{125}I
Half-life ($\times 10^{12}$)	12.43 years	60 days
Mode of decay	Beta	Gamma (Electron capture)
Energy E_{max}	19 keV	Auger electrons
E_{mean}	5.7 keV	35 keV
Detection	Liquid scintillation	Gamma counter
		NaI crystal
Specific activity at 100%	1.07 TBq mA^{-1}	80.5 TBq mA^{-1}
isotopic abundance	28.8 Ci mA^{-1}	2176 Ci mA^{-1}
Daughter nuclide	Helium-3	Tellurium-125

mA (milliatom) = 1/1000 atomic weight in g.

Radiolabeled Immunoassays

41

Table 3. Glossary of other terms related to radioactivity

Alpha (α) emission	Particulate radiation consisting of fast moving helium nuclei
Beta (β) emission	An electron ejected from a nucleus during radioactivity transformation. Beta particles produced by a given nuclide have a range of initial energies from a maximum which is characteristic of the nuclide, down to zero
Carrier-free	A preparation of a radioisotope to which no carrier has been added, and for which precautions have been taken to minimize contamination with other isotopes
Daughter nuclide	Any nuclide that originates from the parent nuclide by radioactive decay
Electron capture	Radioactive transformation in which the nucleus absorbs an electron from an inner orbital. The remaining orbital electrons rearrange to fill the empty electron shell and in so doing energy is released as electromagnetic radiation at X-ray wavelengths and/or as electrons (such electrons are called Auger electrons)
Electron volt (eV)	A unit of energy equal to the kinetic energy required by an electron when accelerated through a potential difference of 1 volt (1 eV = 1.60×10^{12} erg)
Gamma emission	Electromagnetic radiation produced by radioactive decay
Isotopes	Nuclides having the same atomic number but different mass numbers
Isotopic abundance	The number of atoms in a particular isotope in a mixture of the isotopes of an element, expressed as a fraction of all the atoms of the element
Nuclide	A species of atom characterized by its mass number, atomic number and nuclear energy state
Parent nuclide	The radioactive nuclide which disintegrates

Table 4. Radioiodination methods [2]

	Solid-phase lactoperoxidase	Chloramine T	Iodogen
Antigen	0.5–1.0 nmol in minimum volume 0.5 M phosphatase pH 7.4 (e.g. 10 μl)		
Radioiodine	37 MBq (1 mCi) of carrier free ^{125}I-sodium iodide		
Oxidant	0.4 lactoperoxidase coupled to solid-phase with 0.5 nmol H_2O_2 every 10 min	10 μg Chloramine T in minimum volume	50 μl Iodogen dried on surface of reaction tube
Stopping reagent	Phosphate buffer containing sodium azide	10 μg sodium metabisulfide in minimum volume	Dilute reaction with phosphate buffer pH 7.4
Transfer	Use 50 mM phosphate buffer (pH 7.4) containing 1% BSA and 1% potassium iodide		

Radiolabeled Immunoassays

43

Table 5. Methods used for purifying radiolabeled tracers

Method	Salient features	Ref.
1. Column chromatography using gel exclusion		
(i) Sephadex G25	Column 10 × 1 cm; flow rate 3 ml h^{-1}; purifying small radioiodinated molecules <2000 mol. wt	2
(ii) Sephadex G100	Column 60 × 1 cm; flow rate 3 ml h^{-1}; purifying medium size 10–30,000 mol. wt	2
(iii) Sephacryl S300	Column 30 × 1 cm; flow rate 3 ml h^{-1}; purifying large size proteins, e.g. radiolabeled antibodies	4
2. HPLC using ODS	e.g. elution with 50% methanol; flow rate 0.5 ml min^{-1}; columns expensive, use cheaper guard columns	
3. Disposable manual ODS column	ODS loaded into disposable 1 ml syringe with appropriate frits; elution using varying methanol/buffer mixtures; easy to dispose	2
4. TLC	Useful for steroids, drugs, etc. Care required in removing portion of coating containing product; fine dust particles could cause contamination	5
5. Gel electrophoresis using polyacrylamide gels	Exploits difference in charge, particularly relevant to conjugation labels; usually leads to heavy contamination of electrophoresis equipment	6
6. Immunoaffinity chromatography	Micro amounts of immunoadsorbent used in microtubes. Disposable after use. Eluted at low pH, e.g. pH 3 combined with hydrophobic solvent, e.g. 20% acetonitrile	7

Table 6. Glossary of terms related to counting

Background	Caused primarily by cosmic rays and radioactive decay in ground and construction materials 30–40 cpm for ^{125}I
Counting efficiency	Efficiency = (counts per minute/disintegrations per minute) × 100%
Crosstalk	Counts registered in one detector arising from emissions arising from samples in other detectors. This is not a problem with ^{125}I. Usually applies to higher energy isotopes, e.g. ^{57}Co
Crosstalk correction	Adjustment made to counts registered to correct for crosstalk (see above). Extends range of energies measured
Dead time	The time after detected pulse during which the counter is insensitive to next pulse, e.g. 5 μsec. Significant with very high count rates
Efficiency normalization	Adjustment made to counts registered by each detector in a multi-detector counter to effectively eliminate or reduce variation due to different counting efficiencies of the detectors
Energy resolution	Full width of the peak at ½ max, usually as % of main peak energy. Typical for ^{125}I = 25%
Lower limit of detection	= $(3 \times \sqrt{background} (cps))/(efficiency \times volume (liter) \times \sqrt{time} (sec))$
Spillover	Counts registered in one window arising from neighbouring window. Relevant only when counting dual labeled assays at the same time, e.g. ^{57}Co-vitamin B_{12} and ^{125}I-folate, up to 2% if uncorrected
Window	Range of energies instrument is set to detect

Table 7. Units of radiation dose

SI unit of dose	Symbol	Definition	Equivalent old units
Gray (adsorbed dose)	Gy	1 Gy = 10^{-2} joules of energy absorbed per kg of material irradiated	100 rad
Sievert (dose equivalent)	Sv	Measure of absorbed dose and its radiobiological effectiveness (RBE) $Sv = Gy \times Q$ (Q is a constant and for x and g radiation Q = 1)	100 rem (1 rem = $10^{0}mSv$)
Roentgen	R	Measure of x and y radiation expressed in terms of amount of ionization produced in air IR = 2.58×10^{-4} coulombs kg^{-1} air	

Table 8. Annual limits on intake

Isotopee	Annual limits on intake	Derived limits for surface or skin contamination
^{3}H	3 GBq (81 mCi)	300 Bq cm^{-2}
^{125}I	1 MBq (27 μCi)	30 Bq cm^{-2}

Table 9. Regulated laboratory area dose limits

	Supervised	Controlled
Dose equivalent rate	>2.5 Sv h^{-1}	>7.5 Sv h^{-1}
Total amount of radioactivity present		
1. ^{125}I[a]	>1 × 10^8 Bq (2.7 mCi)	>3 × 10^8 Bq (8.1 mCi)
2. ^{3}H[b]	>1 × 10^{10} Bq (270 mCi)	>3 × 10^{10} Bq (810 mCi)

[a] Group III - medium radiotoxicity also includes ^{57}Co.
[b] Group IV - low radioactivity.
N.B. Average radiolabeled immunoassays use <5 μCi of tracer.
10 μCi of ^{125}I-tracer would give dose equivalent rate of 0.15 μSv h^{-1}.

Chapter 6 ENZYME-LABELED IMMUNOASSAY – J. Little

1 Introduction

The high catalytic power and reaction specificity of enzymes makes them ideally suited as tracers for immunoassay. Enzymes were first used as immunoassay labels in the 1960s in immunodiffusion and immunoelectrophoretic techniques, and in immunoenzymatic histological procedures [1–3]. Together with the development of solid phase antibodies and antigens in the early 1970s [4, 5], quantitative assay of soluble antigen and antibody by enzyme-labeled immunoassay (EIA) became a practical alternative to radio-labeled assay (RIA).

In addition to heterogeneous assays, in which antibody bound and free fractions have to be physically separated before quantification, enzymes can be used in homogeneous assays which require no separation. They are of two types:

1. when enzyme-labeled antigen is bound by antibody the activity of the label is modulated (AM), due either to steric hindrance or by a change in the conformation of the enzyme protein [6];
2. large analytes with two (or more) adjacent and distinct epitopes allow a proximal linkage (PL) of two enzymes, one of which generates a substrate for the other. The enzymes are carried separately by two antibodies specific for the two epitopes. A signal is only generated in the presence of the analyte [7].

Homogeneous EIAs are relatively insensitive and are therefore limited to the assay of analytes in high concentration.

2 Desirable properties of enzyme labels

For success as an immunoassay label an enzyme has to

Enzyme-labeled Immunoassay

satisfy a number of basic requirements (*Table 1*). In particular, preparation of the labeled reagent (either antigen or antibody, commonly referred to as conjugate) must be technically simple and reproducible. Alternatively, conjugates must be available commercially at realistic cost. They must be both immunologically and enzymatically active and also stable upon storage. Assay reagents (buffer components, preservatives, etc.) can affect enzyme activity; such effects must be minimal or avoided.

Alkaline phosphatase, horse radish peroxidase and β-galactosidase satisfy the above requirements and are used in the majority of cases. *Table 2* lists some of the enzymes used. An additional requirement of a homogeneous assay system is that the enzymatic activity of the antigen conjugate is strongly influenced when it is complexed with antibody. Conjugates for immunostaining histochemical procedures must be small enough to penetrate fixed tissue specimens.

Basic biochemical information on more commonly used

inactivation of the enzyme will result. *Table 4* lists the factors affecting enzyme label activity.

4 Standard enzymatic assays and activity unit definitions for common enzyme labels

The definition of enzyme activity is based upon the rate of conversion of substrate. The units so assigned are dependent upon the conditions of test procedure which must be described when quoting activity. Generally the concentration of enzyme is such that, as the product is being formed, the concentration of substrate is not significantly altered. The vast majority of standard enzyme assays are spectrophotometric and usually the rate of formation of a chromophore product is measured using the Beer–Lambert law,

$$A = Ecl,$$

where A = absorbance, E = extinction coefficient of product (µmolar), c = concentration (µmol ml^{-1}), l = light path (cm).

enzyme labels is given in *Table 3*. These features have bearing on isolation (cost and availability), conjugation methods, conjugate stability and compatibility with immunoassay systems. Enzymes suitable for use in immunoassay are available commercially (see list of suppliers).

3 Factors affecting function of enzyme labels

Enzymes are biological entities. They are proteins and therefore have limited stability. For an enzyme label to be used optimally in immunoassay suitable conditions have to be complied with both during the immunoassay and when quantifying the label at the conclusion of the procedure. Catalytic activity and stability is dependent on the physicochemical environment (pH, temperature) and on certain requirements such as the presence of metal ions or cofactors. Where activators exist they should be supplied and inhibitors should be avoided. For example, sodium azide, often used as a bacteriostat in laboratory reagents such as buffers and quality control sera, must not come into contact with HRP at any stage because part or complete

Rate of change of product concentration $= dp/dt = A/t \times 1/EI$ (units μmol min^{-1} ml^{-1}, i.e. U ml^{-1}, reaction mixture).

If the concentration of enzyme protein in the reaction mixture is $[E]RM$ mg ml^{-1} then:

$$\text{Specific activity} = A/t \times 1/(EI.[E]RM) \; \text{U mg}^{-1}.$$

For some enzymes there are a number of assay procedures in use (see AP and HRP, *Table 5*) and the worker should verify which system has been used to assign activity, particularly when comparing different preparations. Where a specific activity of an enzyme or enzyme conjugate is quoted the method of protein analysis should also be described, (e.g. Biuret, Lowry dryweight or absorbance at 280 nm, etc).

Table 5 gives details of the activity units of HRP, AP and BG, and *Table 6* of other enzymes used in EIA.

5 Enzyme labeling procedures

There are numerous ways of labeling immunoreactive

biomolecules with enzymes (conjugation). Antibodies, the majority of antigens, and enzymes are all proteins, and, therefore, general methods of protein covalent cross-linking can be adapted to the production of immunoassay reagents [37, 38]. The same chemistries can often be used for conjugating small hapten molecules such as steroids, thyroid hormones and oligopeptides. In the latter, methods may have to be adapted to allow for the properties of the hapten. As a general rule it is desirable to use mild conditions, i.e. aqueous, neutral pH buffers of physiological ionic strength, in order to preserve the maximum activity of the product, commonly referred to as the conjugate).

A number of basic strategies (see *Table 7*) may be employed. Superior products are obtained with heterobifunctional reagents. A variety of water soluble reagents of high reaction specificity are now available commercially. It is desirable to always purchase cross linkers and all chemicals used for conjugation of the highest purity. Enzymes should be of required specific activity (see Section 4) and of high

to link to free sulfhydryls (-SH) present in a second protein or ligand. Where disulfide bridges exist, free -SH may be produced by partial reduction with dithiothreitol (20 mM with EDTA) [37] or, in the case of antibody, with β-mercaptoethylamine. HCl, which does not cause dissociation of heavy and light chains. Reduction may change the conformation and binding activity of biomolecules so, alternatively, free -SH may be introduced via -NH$_2$ using *n*-succinimidyl *s*-acetylthioacetate (SATA) [40] or 2-iminothiolane. HCl (Trauts reagent) [41]. SATA is preferred because introduced -SH are protected preventing dimerization. When required for conjugation -SH is exposed by deacylation with aqueous hydroxylamine (50 mM, pH 7.5 with Na$_2$HPO$_4$ with 2.5 mM EDTA).

Aldehydes react with primary amine under mildly alkaline and reducing conditions forming a peptide bond via a Schiff base intermediate [42]. Periodate oxidation of glycoprotein carbohydrate, containing vicinal hydroxyls, produces reactive endogenous aldehyde (see *Table 8*).

purity (check specifications of commercial suppliers). Clean glassware should be used, particularly when using organic solvents. For optimal assay performance careful purification and storage of the conjugate is necessary.

5.1 Standard conjugation methodology

Maximum yields require optimization but products suitable for use in immunoassay can be obtained using the reaction schemes below as a guide.

N-hydroxysuccinimide esters react with primary amino groups present in proteins or ligand to be conjugated at slightly alkaline pH (50 mM sodium phosphate, pH 7.5 containing 1 mM EDTA or 50 mM sodium bicarbonate). The reaction produces an amide bond and n-hydroxysuccinimide. Wasteful hydrolysis of the reactive ester (half-life 5 h) [39] is minimized by keeping the concentration of amine high (e.g. IgG at 20 mg ml^{-1}).

Maleimides, pyridyl disulfides and organic halides are used

5.2 Purification of conjugates

For good results in solid phase EIA and IEMA it is always necessary to purify antibody and antigen conjugates. As a general rule the more homogeneous an enzyme labeled reagent then the better it is. The presence of free antibody or hapten will reduce assay sensitivity; large amounts of free enzyme will raise 'background' and thereby reduce precision overall; large polymers or aggregated conjugate will lead to high 'backgrounds' and imprecision. Polymerized conjugate can be avoided and free enzyme and antibody is minimized by using an appropriate conjugation chemistry.

Following conjugation the purification strategy is as follows:

For antibody

1. remove conjugate from unreacted enzyme;
2. remove unreacted antibody from conjugate.

For hapten

1. remove conjugate from unreacted hapten;
2. remove unreacted enzyme from conjugate (often not required).

Enzyme-labeled Immunoassay

6 Reporting systems for EIA

Detection and quantification of an enzyme label is usually achieved by following a chemical conversion. A detailed knowledge of enzyme kinetics is unnecessary for immunoassay applications. It is possible to select a suitable reporting system from a range of published standard methods, each optimal for a type of assay format. There are three main types of detection technology:

1. spectrophotometric (colorimetric) in which the absorbance of a product is followed;
2. fluorometric in which the appearance of a fluorescent product is followed (see Chapter 7);
3. chemiluminescent in which light produced by a chemical reaction, catalyzed by the enzyme, is measured (see Chapter 8).

In the case of immunostaining an insoluble colored or fluorescent product is desirable. In solid-phase assays, such as coated test tubes or microtiter wells, a soluble chromophore or fluorophore product is required.

6.1 Spectrophotometric systems

A chromophore product is formed from a chromogenic substrate by action of the enzyme label. The product is monitored photometrically, usually by means of specialized equipment, such as tube or microplate readers. The absorbance (response) is related to analyte concentration using standards or positive/negative controls (see Chapter 11). Details of substrates (including in the case of HRP chromogenic H-donors) are summarized in *Table 9*.

Often the enzymatic reaction is terminated with a 'stopping' reagent, such as sulfuric acid. The chromophore absorbtion spectrum may change with stopping reagent; ensure readings are made at the correct wavelength. Stopping is not essential when using modern automated equipment, such as microplate readers, as the reading time is very short (e.g. 5 seconds).

Instead of stopped or 'end-point' determinations, kinetic readings may be employed. Linear rate of change of absorbance is computed and used as the response.

In addition to physicochemical detection enzymes are able to generate electromotive potential (see Chapter 10).

In addition to simple substrates enzyme amplification systems (pioneered by IQ Bio [56]) may be used with the primary enzyme label (mainly AP).

Table 1. Qualitative requirements of enzyme labels

1. Enzyme should be commercially available and affordable and/or able to be prepared simply in the laboratory
2. High molar activity – a single enzyme molecule is capable of generating many product molecules from substrate in a given time[a]
3. Labeling of reagent is simple, producing reproducible and characterizable conjugates
4. Conjugates are stable or can be stabilized and can be stored without deterioration
5. Conjugate enzymatic activity can be readily measured[b] and is resistant to interference by either assay components or factors[c] which may be present in specimens

[a]SI unit the katal, 1 mol substrate per second. Previously expressed as the turnover number (TN), units mol per min per catalytic site.
[b]By a reproducible and robust assay, zero order kinetics, negligible product inhibition.
[c]Inhibitors, anti-enzyme antibodies, endogenous enzyme, substrate analogs.

Enzyme-labeled Immunoassay

Table 2. Enzyme labels for immunoassay

Enzyme – recommended name[a]	Systematic name[a]	Enzyme commission number[a]	Separation assays IA[b]/IMA[c]	Homogenous assays AM[d]/PL[e]	Immuno-staining IH[f]/WB[g]
Horse radish peroxidase (HRP)	Donor:hydrogen-peroxidase oxidoreductase	EC 1.11.1.7	IA, IMA	PL (with GO)	IH, WB
Alkaline phosphatase (AP)	Orthophosphoric-monoester phosphohydrolase	EC 3.1.3.1	IA, IMA		IH, WB
β-Galactosidase (BG)	β-D-Galactoside galactohydrolase	EC 3.2.1.23	IA, IMA		
Glucose oxidase (GO)	β-D-Glucose:oxygen 1-oxidoreductase	EC 1.1.3.4	IA, IMA	PL (with HRP)	IH, WB
Urease	Urea amidohydrolase	EC 3.5.1.5	IA, IMA		
Malate dehydrogenase (MDH)	Malate:NAD$^+$ oxidoreductase	EC 1.1.1.37		AM	
Glucose-6-phosphate dehydrogenase (GPD)	D-Glucose-6-phosphate:NAD(P)$^+$ 1 oxidoreductase	EC 1.1.1.49		AM, PL (with HK)	
Hexokinase (HK)	ATP:D-hexose 6-phosphotransferase	EC 2.7.1.1		PL (with GDP)	
Carbonic anhydrase (CA)	Carbonate dehydratase	EC 4.2.1.1	IA, IMA	AM	
Lysozyme	Peptidogycan N-acetylmuramoylhydrolase	EC 3.2.1.17			
Glucoamylase		EC 3.2.1.3	IA, IMA		
Microperoxidase (MP)	–				IH
Ribonuclease A	Ribonucleate 3'-pyrimidino-oligonucleotidohydrolase	EC 3.1.27.5		AM	
Pyrophosphatase (PP)		EC 3.6.1.1	IMA		
β-Lactamase	Penicillin amido-β-lactam hydrolase	EC 3.5.2.6	IA		
Acetylcholinesterase	Acetylcholine acetylhydrolase	EC 3.1.1.7	IA, IMA		

[a]Systematic classification according to recommendations of the Enzyme Commission [8]. [b]IA, limited antibody, competitive immunoassay. [c]IMA, excess antibody, immunometric assay. [d]AM, activity modulation. [e]PL, proximal linkage. [f]IH, immunohistochemistry. [g]WB, western blot. Note: luciferase has been used infrequently.

Table 3. Biochemical properties of important enzyme labels

Enzyme	Source	Monomeric molecular mass (da)	Protein structure	Carbohydrate content (mass %)	$E^{1\%}_{280nm}$	pI	Ref.
HRP (isozyme c)	Horse radish roots, Amoracia rusticana	44 000	308 amino acids, 4 disulfide bridges, monomeric	22	6.7	8.7	9
AP	Bovine intestinal mucosa	84 500	Dimeric active species		10	5.7	10, 11
AP	E. coli	80 000	Globular, dimeric active species		7.2	4.5	12
BG	E. coli	116 250	Tetramer plus larger aggregates			4.6	13
GO	Aspergillus niger	76 500	Dimer, globular	12	18	4.3	14
Urease	Jack bean Canavalia ensiformis	480 000			7		15
Lysozyme	Egg white	14 600	Each monomer 129 amino acids, 4 disulfide bonds, mainly dimeric		25.5	11	16
MDH	Porcine heart mitochondria	35 000	Dimeric			6.2	17
GPD	Leuconostoc mesenteroides	52 000	Dimeric				18
8-MP[a]	Proteolysis of horse heart cytochrome c	1502 (8-MP)	8, 9 and 11 amino acids with heme			4.9	19
9-MP[a]		1630 (9-MP)					
11-MP[a]		1857 (11-MP)					

[a]Number indicates length of peptide.

Enzyme-labeled Immunoassay

Table 4. Factors affecting enzyme label activity

Enzyme	Substrate	K_M[a]	pH optimum	Activators	Inhibitors	Metal, coenzyme* or prosthetic group**	Ref.
HRP (isozyme c)	Hydrogen peroxide	N-A	6–7		NaN_3 > 10^{-3} M, O_2, Cl_2, Fl_2, hydroxylamine, styrene, CN^- > 10^{-6} M, S^{2-} > 10^{-6} M, hydroxymethylhydrogen peroxide [b]	Protohematin IX**	20, 21
AP (bacterial and bovine)	Phosphate esters		8–10	1 mM Mg^{2+}, 0.1 mM Zn^{2+}, diethanolamine[c]	Inorganic phosphate > 50 μM[d,e], arsenate[d], chelating agents[f], amino acids[d,g]	Zn^{2+}, two per subunit	9, 22, 23
BG	D-Galactopyranosides	3.9 mM (lactose)	7.2–7.7	1 mM Mg^{2+}	β-Mercatoethanol alone, mercurials alone		13
GO	β-D-Glucose/oxygen	28 mM/ 0.18 mM	5–6		p-Chloromercuribenzoate, nitrate, 8-hydroxyquinoline, D-arabinose, 2-deoxy-D-glucose	FAD*, one per subunit	12, 24
Urease	Urea	10.3 mM	4.8	Inorganic phosphate	Univalent cations		13, 25
GPD (bacterial)	Glucose-6-phosphate		7.8	Mg^{2+} < 10 mM	Divalent cations, phosphate	NAD^+, one per subunit	18, 26
MDH	Oxaloacetic acid	0.045 mM	7.4	Phosphate, arsenate, Zn^{2+}, malate	Oxaloacetate, 8-hydroxyquinoline, phenols, sulfite	NAD^+, one per subunit	27

[a]Applicable where an enzyme obeys Michaelis–Menten theory. [b]Although inhibition may be reversible all should be avoided. [c]See specific enzymatic assay details. [d]Competitive. [e]Uncompetitive. [f]EDTA, EGTA, cysteine. [g]Inorganic phosphate may be present in substrate preparations.

Table 5. Activity units of HRP, AP and BG

Enzyme	Unit definition	Assay detail	Specific activity suitable for EIA (U mg^{-1})	Ref.
AP	*Method 1*[a]: That amount of enzyme causing the hydrolysis of one micromole of p-nitrophenyl phosphate (PNP) per minute at pH 9.6 and 25°C	PNP + H$_2$O → p-nitrophenol + H$_3$PO$_4$ Reaction with 4.4 mM PNP in 25 mM glycine, pH 9.6 / 8.3 mM MgCl$_2$. E_{405nm}^{mM} = 18.7	> 2000	28
AP	*Method 2*[a]: That amount of enzyme causing the hydrolysis of one μmol of PNP per minute at pH 9.8 and 37°C in the presence of diethanolamine	Reaction with 10 mM p-nitrophenylphosphate in 1.0 M diethanolamine, pH 9.8 / 0.5 mM MgCl$_2$. E_{405nm}^{M} = 18.2	> 7000	29
HRP[b]	*Guaiacol assay*: That amount of enzyme which causes the conversion of one micromole of hydrogen peroxide per minute at 25°C	H$_2$O$_2$ + DH$_2$ → 2H$_2$O + D 0.333 mM guaiacol in 100 mM potassium phosphate, pH 7.0. Reaction initiated with 0.13 mM H$_2$O$_2$[c]. $E_{436nm}^{μM}$ = 25.5	> 200	15
HRP	*Pyrogallol assay*[d]: One unit[e] of HRP will produce 1 mg purpurogallin from pyrogallol in 20 sec at pH 6.0 and 20°C	0.533% (w/v) pyrogallol, 10 mM sodium phosphate pH 6.0, 8 mM H$_2$O$_2$. Specific activity = $\frac{(A_{420}/20sec)}{12 \times [HRP]}$	> 300	30
HRP	*ABTS®* assay: Unit as guaiacol assay	8.65 mM 2,2′-azino-di(3-ethylbenzothiazoline-6-sulfonate) (ABTS®) in 100 mM potassium phosphate. Reaction initiated with 0.3 mM H$_2$O$_2$. $E_{405nm}^{μM}$ = 36.8	> 200	31

continued

57   *Enzyme-labeled Immunoassay*

Table 5. Activity units of HRP, AP and BG, *continued*

Enzyme	Unit definition	Assay detail	Specific activity suitable for EIA (U mg^{-1})	Ref.
BG	That amount of enzyme which causes the hydrolysis of 1 mol of o-nitrophenylgalactopyranoside (NPG) per minute at 37°C, pH 7.8[f]	Reaction of 2.7 mM NPG in 50 mM potassium phosphate, pH 7.8/1 mM MgCl$_2$/10 mM β-mercaptoethanol. $E_{405nm}^{\mu M} = 3.5$	> 800	32

[a]Units obtained with method 2 approx 3.3 times those with method 1.

[b]Reinheitzhal (R_z), the ratio of A_{403} to A_{280}, is a measure of HRP hemin to protein content. Pure isoenzyme C has an R_z around 3.5. R_z is not a guarantee of specific activity.

[c]Check H$_2$O$_2$ conc: 8 mM (0.025%) solution in dH$_2$O A$_{240}$ = 0.35.

[d]Pyrogallol method used by Sigma has been largely replaced by the Guaiacol.

[e]Approx 18 mol min^{-1} at 25°C.

[f]Use a reference BG preparation to check recovery. Alternative substrates include 4-NPG and a lactose substrate/galactose dehydrogenase coupled assay following NADH formation.

See references for specific assay details.

Table 6. Units of infrequently used enzyme labels

Enzyme	Unit definition	Assay details	Specific activity suitable for immunoassay	Ref.
GO	Amount of enzyme which causes oxidation of one micromole glucose per minute at 25°C, pH 7.0	D-Glucose + O_2 + H_2O → D-gluconolactone + H_2O_2 Peroxide detected by coupled HRP assay. o-Dianisidine dihydrochloride hydrogen donor; $E_{340nm}^{\mu M} = 8.3$	360	15
MDH	Amount of enzyme causing the oxidation of one micromole of NADH per minute at 25°C and pH 7.4	Oxaloacetate + NADH + H^+ → (S)-malate + NAD^+ Rate of disappearance of NADH followed at 340nm; $E_{340nm}^{\mu M} = 6.22$	1500	33
GPD *L. mesenteroides*	Amount of enzyme causing the reduction of one micromole of NAD^+ per minute at 25°C and pH 7.8	D-Glucose-6-phosphate + NAD^+ → 6-glucono-1,5-lactone 6-phosphate + NADH + H^+ Appearance of NADH monitored spectrophotometrically	500	34
Urease	Amount of enzyme which liberates one micromole of ammonia per minute at 25°C and pH 7.0	Urea + H_2O → CO_2 + $2NH_3$ Following incubation with substrate NH_3 liberation detected with Nessler's reagent	1400	35
Lysozyme	Amount of enzyme causing a decrease in extinction of 0.001 per minute at 450 nm, 25°C and pH 6.24 of *Micrococcus lysodeikticus*	Lysis of a suspension (0.25 mg ml^{-1}, A = 1.3, λ = 450 nm) of *M. lysodeikticus*. Due to the biological nature of the substrate a reference preparation should be used	1500	36

Enzyme-labeled Immunoassay

Table 7. Strategies of conjugation

Method	Strategy	Advantages	Disadvantages	Example
Via existing molecular structures	To use chemical moieties present on the biomolecule as a handle for linkage. They may be activated chemically, e.g. oxidation	Minimal modification of the native molecule	Often heterogeneous, uncharacterized products	Periodate oxidation of carbohydrate
One-step reaction	All molecules (enzyme, immunoreagent and linker, if used) reacted simultaneously	Simple protocol. Conjugates suited to immunohistochemistry (IH)	Immunological inactivation (large aggregates), formation of homopolymers, high assay blanks	N/A
Two-step reaction	One molecule activated or exposed to a reactive linker in excess, isolated then reacted with the second	Aggregation avoided. Superior characterization of products	Formation of homopolymers	N/A
Homo-bifunctional reagent	A chemical linker which carries two identical functions reactive to groups on the immunoreagents	May be used in one- and two-step methods. Simple protocols	Formation of homopolymers and high orders of conjugation-heterogeneous product. often limited aqueous solubility	Glutaraldehyde (GA)
Hetero-bifunctional reagent	A chemical linker with two different functions reactive to different groups on the immunoreagents	May be used in one- and two-step protocols. With appropriate selection homopolymers, higher orders of conjugation can be avoided. Well characterized and reproducible products	Often limited aqueous solubility	Succinimidyl 4-(N-maleimido-methyl) cyclohexane-1-carboxylate (SMCC)

| Non-immunological ligand-binder | Ligand and binder (other than antigen:antibody) combined separately with one of the immunoreagents and the enzyme. Enzyme labeling achieved by bringing the two together | | |
| Avidin–biotin, streptavidin–biotin[a] | A multipurpose modified enzyme reagent (e.g. streptavidin-enzyme) can be used in all assay systems where the complimentary immunoreagent (biotinyl-antigen or -antibody) exists. Alternatively, different streptavidin-enzyme may be used | Despite claims of the possibility of higher ratios of enzyme to immunoreagent poorer sensitivity due to raised nonspecific binding | 43 |

[a]See also Chapter 2.

Table 8. Conjugation reaction conditions

Method	Use of reagent	Ref.
Periodate	Oxidize glycoprotein[a] at 5 mg ml^{-1} in 0.1 M $NaHCO_3$ with 4 mM $NaIO_4$ for 2h at 20°C. Remove oxidizing agent and add second molecule (containing $-NH_3$) in molar ratio of 1:1.5[b] in $NaHCO_3$/5 mM $NaCNBH_3$	43
SMCC[c]	100 mg of SMCC at 10 mg ml^{-1} in DMF to 5 mg protein; reacted for 2h at 4°C. Remove unreacted reagent and add second molecule containing $-SH$[d], molar ratio 1:1, and incubate 2 h at 20°C	44
GA (two step)	Activate 5 mg enzyme with 10 ml GA[e] for 18 h at 20°C. Remove excess GA and add second molecule (containing $-NH_3$) at molar ratio of 4:1 in 0.1 M $NaCO_3$/5 mM $NaCNBH_3$ and react for 24 h at 20°C	45

[a]e.g. HRP. [b]e.g. antibody; increase up to 10-fold excess for haptens with one $-NH^3$ per molecule. [c]Can substitute other heterobifunctional reagents. [d]If not endogenous introduce with SATA. [e]Monomer.

Table 9. Commonly used chromogenic substrates for enzyme-labeled immunoassay

Enzyme label	Substrate	Acronym	Product[a]	Ref.
AP	*p*-Nitrophenyl phosphate	PNP	S	46
AP	Phenolphthalein monophosphate[b]	PMP	S	47
AP	5-Bromo-4-chloro-3-indolyl phosphate/nitro blue tetrazolium	BCIP/NBT	IS	48
HRP	3,3',5,5'-Tetramethylbenzidine[b]	TMB	S	49
HRP	*o*-Phenylenediamine	OPD	S	50
HRP	*o*-Dianisidine	–	S	51
HRP	2,2'-Azino-bis(3-ethylbenzthiazoline-6-sulphonic acid)	ABTS[R]	S	52
HRP	5-Aminosalicylic acid	5AS	S	53
HRP	3,3'-Diaminobenzidine	DAB	IS	54
HRP	3-Amino-9-ethylcarbazole	AEC	IS	55
BG	2-Nitrophenol-b-D-galactopyranoside[b]	NPDG	S	55

[a] S = soluble product, suitable for solid phase EIA and IEMA (ELISA); IS = insoluble product, suitable for IH and WB purposes.

[b] Recommended for sensitive EIA and IEMA.

[c] Reaction stopped with 0.5 M H_2SO_4 final concentration.

[d] *Care in use!* mutagenic or carcinogenic.

[e] Reaction may be terminated with cyanide (5 mM final concentration). *Care!*

Chapter 7 FLUORESCENT AND PHOSPHORESCENT LABELED ASSAYS – S. Blincko

1 Introduction

The use of photoluminescent (fluorescent and phosphorescent) compounds in immunoassays has now become routine. The problems of sensitivity due the high background fluorescence of serum have been overcome by the use of lanthanide chelates with time-resolved detection [1–3] or by the use of enzymes which convert nonfluorescent substrates to fluorescent products (e.g. alkaline phosphatase and 4-methylumbelliferone phosphate). Many other assays have been developed that do not require such great sensitivity, with fluorescein derivatives being the most common label (e.g. polarization fluoroimmunoassay (PFIA)). There remains a vast wealth of technology that has not yet been exploited to its full potential. Some nonseparation assays (other than PFIA) may become more widely used (e.g. fluorescence quenching techniques). This chapter reviews the strategies employed in photoluminescent immunoassays (see *Table 1*), the compounds that have been, or potentially may be, employed in photoluminescent assays and the practical methods for performing such assays.

2 Photoluminescence

When a molecule absorbs light of sufficient energy it attains an electronically excited state. If the process of relaxation from the excited state back to the ground state includes the emission of light, it is called photoluminescence. Fluorescence is photoluminescence where the light emissive transition involves electronic states of the same multiplicity (e.g. singlet–singlet). Phosphorescence, by contrast, is photoluminescence where the light emissive transition involves states of differing multiplicity (e.g. triplet–singlet).

Fluorescent and Phosphorescent Labeled Assays

the centre of the sample is diminished (inner filter effect) and so the emission is also diminished. To overcome this, front-face (front-surface) measurements are employed.

4 Photoluminescent compounds

A number of fluorescent and phosphorescent compounds are employed in immunoassays. The photophysical properties of compounds that are used in immunoassay and many others that may find application are described in *Tables 2 and 3*. The photophysical properties are characterized by the following terms:

λ_{ex}, the excitation maximum wavelength (nm);
λ_{em}, the emission maximum wavelength (nm);
Stokes' shift, the difference between the excitation and emission wavelengths (nm). This figure does not take into account the breadth of the excitation and emission peaks. It is safe to assume that all peaks are broad except those from

The wavelength of the emitted light is always longer than the exciting light (Stokes' law) and the Stokes' shift is defined as the difference between the excitation and emission wavelengths.

The ratio of the number of photons absorbed and the excitation wavelength to those emitted is the quantum yield. This is expressed as a decimal fraction of 1 and gives a measure of the efficiency of the process leading to light emission. As important as quantum yield is the extinction coefficient of the compound at the excitation wavelength. For a strong luminescent signal the quantum yield and the extinction coefficient should be high.

The lifetime of the emission may be measured and varies from 10^{-9} to 10^{-1} sec.

3 Fluorimetry

There are three main methods of fluorimetry currently employed for immunoassays:

1. conventional: continuous excitation source with continuous detection;
2. time-resolved: pulses of excitation light followed by a time delay before detection. This method is only appropriate for compounds with long fluorescent lifetimes (e.g. lanthanide chelates) and allows the short lifetime background fluorescence to diminish, so improving the signal to noise ratio;
3. polarization: polarized excitation source with the emission read parallel and perpendicular to the plane of polarization.

A wide range of fluorimeters are available from commercial sources using cells, tubes or flow cells as sample holders. There are also dedicated plate readers to take 96-well microtiter plates (clear, black or white plastic) or clear microtiter strips.

Fluorescence measurement of dilute solutions is isotropic. However, at high absorbance the intensity of light reaching

the emission of the lanthanide chelates [3];

φ, the quantum yield of photoluminescence;

τ, the lifetime of the emission (nsec);

ε, the molar extinction coefficient at the excitation wavelength ($cm^{-1} M^{-1}$).

The optimum properties for use in immunoassay are a high extinction coefficient and quantum yield, a large Stokes' shift (> 50 nm) and an emission wavelength greater than 500 nm, preferably greater than 600 nm (to be clear of the fluorescence of proteins etc. in serum). Tables 2 and 3 detail the photophysical properties of a wide range of luminescent compounds. Some are used in immunoassays while others are included to give a choice for new applications. The inclusion of ovalbumin and gamma globulin conjugate data is to enable the properties of protein conjugates to be compared with the reactive compound. Ovalbumin was chosen as it has both free thiol and amine groups. In many cases quantum yields drop on conjugation to proteins [14].

Fluorescent and Phosphorescent Labeled Assays

5 Preparation of photoluminescent labels

Table 4 shows the reactive groups for coupling of fluorochromes to antibodies and proteins.

Aromatic diazonium salts are not recommended for coupling fluorophores to proteins because the product is usually very weakly fluorescent.

For fluorophores derivatized to couple to other functional groups see the *Molecular Probes Handbook of Fluorescent Probes and Research Chemicals* [15], *Fluorescent Protein Conjugates* [24] and *Covalent Fluorescent Probes* [23].

5.1 The conditions for coupling fluorochromes to antibodies and proteins

The main problem encountered is overlabeling which has two effects:

1. self quenching of the fluorophore; above a certain number of fluorescent molecules (typically 10) coupled to the one antibody molecule the fluorescence does not increase but decreases (this does not apply to the lanthanide labels);

2. reduction of the binding activity of the antibody; this varies among different antibody preparations and so has to be optimized each time.

Table 5 describes the reaction conditions used and *Table 6* specific labeling procedures.

6 Background fluorescence

Background fluorescence (see *Table 7*) is often a limitation on the efficacy of immunoassays using fluorescent-labeled tracers, particularly those used in the measurement of complex biological specimens.

Table 1. Strategies for immunoassay employing photoluminescent labels

Method	Comment	Detection method
FIA	Sensitivity of fluorescein labeled assays down to ~ 1 nmol⁻¹. Dissociation enhanced luminescence fluoroimmunoassay (DELFIA) method is more sensitive and has found wide application [1–3]	DELFIA [3] by time-resolved fluorimetry. Other labels by conventional fluorimetry
IFMA	Sensitivity of fluorescein labeled assays down to ~ 1 nmol⁻¹. DELFIA method is more sensitive and has found wide application [1–3]	DELFIA [3] by time-resolved fluorimetry. Other labels by conventional fluorimetry
PFIA	Nonseparation FIA where the intensity of the polarized fluorescence increases when the labeled hapten binds to antibody. Simple and rapid – ideal for most haptens. It has found particular application for therapeutic drug monitoring and drugs of abuse screening. Sensitivity of fluorescein labeled assays down to ~ 0.1 µmol l⁻¹. Suitable for molecules below 20 000 da	Fluorescence polarization detection
Enzyme immunoassays (EIA and IEMA) with nonfluorescent substrates that are converted to fluorescent products	The nonfluorescent substrates are converted to fluorescent products. The use of alkaline phosphatase as label to convert 4-methylumbelliferone phosphate (nonfluorescent) to 4-methylumbelliferone is widely used and gives greater sensitivity than enzyme-labeled methods with colorimetric substrates	Conventional fluorimetry
Fluorescence quenching immunoassay (nonseparation)	FIA where the intensity of the fluorescence decreases when the labeled hapten binds to antibody. Not universally applicable to all haptens [4–7]	Time-resolved and conventional fluorimetry

Fluorescent and Phosphorescent Labeled Assays

continued

67

Table 1. Strategies for immunoassay employing photoluminescent labels, *continued*

Method	Comment	Detection method
Fluorescence enhancement immunoassay (nonseparation)	FIA where the intensity of the fluorescence increases when the labeled hapten binds to antibody. Potentially useful for haptens which quench fluorescence [8]	Conventional fluorimetry
Fluorescence energy transfer immunoassay (nonseparation)	Fluorophore labeled antigen and quencher labeled antibody. The addition of unlabeled antigen reduces the quenching [9–10]	Conventional fluorimetry
Phosphoroimmunoassays (separation and nonseparation)	FIA with phosphorescent label [4]	Time-resolved fluorimetry
Alternative binding immunoassays (nonseparation)	Immune complexes of anti-fluorescein and anti-hapten antibodies are formed. The FITC-hapten label may bind to antibodies of either specificity but not at the same time. Binding to anti-fluorescein markedly quenches the fluorescence, whereas binding to anti-hapten did not. Addition of unlabeled hapten results in more label binding to anti-fluorescein and so diminishes the fluorescence signal [11]	Conventional fluorimetry
Fluorescence protection immunoassay or indirect quenching immunoassay (nonseparation)	FIA for some proteins where antibodies to fluorescein will bind to, and quench, the fluorescence of the free fraction but not the bound [12, 13]	Conventional fluorimetry

DELFIA, dissociation enhanced luminescence fluoroimmunoassay.

The method employs antigen or antibody labeled with a lanthanide chelate complex. The complex is not highly fluorescent but is stable in basic solutions. After the final separation step of the assay an enhancement solution is added. This acidic solution releases the lanthanide ion into solution where it combines with a chelating agent and forms a highly fluorescent complex. This complex is stabilized by the detergent tri-*n*-octylphosphine oxide (TOPO) added in the enhancement solution.

Table 2. Photoluminescent compounds

Name	λ,ex (nm)	λ,em (nm)	Stokes' shift (nm)	ϕ	ε (cm^{-1}M^{-1})	τ (nsec)	Solvent	Refs/notes
B-Phycoerythrin	546,565	575	29,10	0.98	2.41×10^6		Aqueous	9, 15, 16
R-Phycoerythrin	480,546, 565	578	98,32,13	0.82	1.96×10^6		Aqueous	9, 15, 16
Allophycocyanin	650	660	10	0.68	0.7×10^6		Aqueous	9, 15, 16
Fluorescein isothiocyanate	492	517	25	~0.9	76 000	3.8	pH 9.0 (emission intensity drops below pH 9.0)	14, 15 Quantum yield drops on conjugation to protein
Fluorescein isothiocyanate–ovalbumin conjugate	490	525	35	~0.85		3.7	pH 7.4	17
Fluorescein isothiocyanate–gamma globulin conjugate	495	525	30	~0.5		4.2	pH 9.0	14
Fluorescein-5-maleimide	490	515	25		83 000		pH 9.0	15 Spectrum of mercapto-ethanol derivative
Rhodamine B isothiocyanate–protein conjugate	550	585	35	~0.7		3.0	pH 7.4	18
Tetramethylrhodamine-5-isothiocyanate	544	570	26		100 000		Methanol	15

continued

69   *Fluorescent and Phosphorescent Labeled Assays*

Table 2. Photoluminescent compounds, *continued*

Name	λex (nm)	λem (nm)	Stokes' shift (nm)	φ	ε (cm⁻¹M⁻¹)	τ (nsec)	Solvent	Refs/notes
Tetramethylrhodamine-5-isothiocyanate–ovalbumin conjugate	546	582	36			2.3	pH 7.4	17
Tetramethylrhodamine-5-isothiocyanate–gamma globulin conjugate	550	580	30	~0.7		~3	pH 8.0	14
Texas Red (sulfonyl chloride)	589	615	26		85 000		Methanol	15 Spectrum of butylamine derivative
Dansyl chloride (sulfonyl chloride)	335	578	243	0.06	4600	<15	Water	15 Spectrum of butylamine derivative
Dansyl chloride–ovalbumin conjugate	340	535	95			14	pH 7.4	17
Lucifer Yellow (hydrazide, ammonium salt)	428	533	105		12 000		Water	15
Lucifer Yellow CH–ovalbumin conjugate	419	538	119			7.4	pH 7.4	17
β-Methylumbelliferone-3-acetic acid (N-hydroxysuccinimide ester)	390	460	70		17 000		pH 8.5	15 Spectrum of amine conjugate

τ (nsec) values as listed in column.

Fluorescamine (fluoram)	383	478	95	0.23	7300	7.5	Ethanol	15 Spectrum of butylamine derivative
Fluorescamine–ovalbumin conjugate	370	488	118			6.9	pH 7.4	17
NBD chloride (4-chloro-7-nitrobenzo-2-oxa-1,3-diazole)-ovalbumin conjugate	470	544	74			3.2	pH 7.4	17
Cascade blue (acyl azide)	375,396	410	35,14		29 000		Water	15
Pyrene butyric acid	341	377,395	36,54		40 000	~110	Methanol	15
Europium (2-napthoyltrifluoroacetone)$_3^{3+}$	340	613	273	0.69	36 000	730 000	Acidic buffer	3 Standard DELFIA reagents (included Triton X-100, and TOPO)
Samarium (2-naphthoyltrifluoroacetone)$_3^{3+}$	340	643	303	0.02	36 000	50 000	Acidic buffer	3 As above
Terbium^{3+} (Diethylenetriamine-pentacetic acid anhydride-4-aminosalicylic acid-serum albumin conjugate)	312	545	233			1 580 000	Basic buffer	19, 20 No dissociation required. Potentially useful for nonseparation assays

continued

Fluorescent and Phosphorescent Labeled Assays

71

Table 2. Photoluminescent compounds, *continued*

Name	λex (nm)	λem (nm)	Stokes' shift (nm)	φ	ε (cm⁻¹M⁻¹)	τ (nsec)	Solvent	Refs/notes
Europium-activated yttrium oxysulfide particle (0.1–0.3 µm)	360	620	260	0.12		760 000		21 Protein A or other proteins coated onto particle surface. Luminescence minimally effected by pH or temperature
Zinc silicate activated with manganese and arsenic	360	522	162			11 ms		21 As above
Eosin-5-isothiocyanate	522	543	21		100 000		pH 9.0	15
Erythrosin-5-isothiocyanate	528	553F 690P	25F 162P	0.002P	86 000	350 000	pH 9.0	4,15 Emission both fluorescent (F) and phosphorescent (P).
Ruthenium(phenanthroline)₂(4,7-diphenylphenanthroline disulphonylchloride)²⁺ .2Cl⁻–IgG conjugate	470	630	160			1200	pH 7.4	22 Potentially useful for time-resolution with laser excitation

For other labels see refs 1–3, 15, 24.

Table 3. Enzymes and their substrates with fluorescent products

Reaction product	λex (nm)	λem (nm)	Stokes' shift (nm)	φ	ε (cm^{-1} M^{-1})	Solution	Enzyme/substrate	Refs/notes
4-Methylumbelliferone	360	450	90		17 000	pH 9.0	Alkaline phosphatase + 4-methylumbelliferone phosphate or β-galactosidase + 4-methylumbelliferyl-β-D-galactopyranoside [15]	The method most commonly used in immunoassays
Fluorescein	490	514	24	~0.9	90 000	pH 9.0	β-galactosidase + fluorescein mono-β-D-galactoside or Alkaline phosphatase + fluorescein diphosphate	13, 25

Table 4. Reactive groups for coupling of fluorochromes to antibodies and proteins

Functional group	Proteins in which group is found	Reactive groups on fluorophores for covalent coupling
NH$_2$	All lysine containing peptides\proteins, free N-terminal amines. e.g. IgG, Fab fragments	Active esters, isothiocyanates, isocyanates, sulfonyl halides, triazines, imidoesters, acyl azides, mixed anhydrides, epoxides, vinyl sulfones
SH	All free thiol containing peptides\proteins (e.g. Fab') and those derivatized by Traut's reagent (2-iminothiolane hydrochloride)	Maleimides, haloacetals, acryloyls, aromatic methyl bromides, pyridyl disulfides

Fluorescent and Phosphorescent Labeled Assays

73

Table 5. Reaction conditions for coupling fluorochromes to antibodies and proteins

Reaction conditions	Comments
Labeling ratio (molar)	Typically 10 mol label to 1 mol antibody. Many fluorophores are impure so this needs to be taken into account [26]. For the lanthanide chelates see labeling procedures below
pH and buffers	Typically pH 9.0 carbonate\bicarbonate for proteins that isothiocyanates and active esters are being added to. By lowering the pH overlabeling or loss of antibody activity may be prevented. Buffers should not contain reagents that react with the labeling compound (e.g. azide, amines and proteins)
Temperature	Typically ambient. May be lowered to 4°C to slow reaction. Temperature has a marked effect on the ratio of labeling achieved for the lanthanide chelate derivatives see labeling procedures below
Time	Typically 2 h. By shortening the reaction time overlabeling or loss of antibody activity may be prevented
Solvent for label	Water is best. However DMF and DMSO may be used provided the final reaction mixture does not exceed 1:10 organic solvent:aqueous buffer. N.B. Proteins other than antibodies may not tolerate as much DMF or DMSO. Where organic solvents cannot be used adsorption of the fluorphore in organic solvent onto celite followed by evaporation and addition to the aqueous solution may be used [23]

Ref. 25 gives many useful details for antibody and F(ab)$_2$ purification and conjugation with fluorophores. Ref. 23 gives a review of labeling methods and conditions.

Table 6. Specific labeling procedures

Product	Method	Ref.
Fluorescein–IgG	React fluorescein isothiocyanate with purified IgG (10:1 molar ratio) in bicarbonate buffer pH 9.0. Purify on Sephadex column	27
Fluorescein–hapten	React fluorescein isothiocyanite with amino-derivatized hapten in methanol. Purify on TLC	28
Eu chelate–IgG	React derivatized Eu chelate with purified IgG overnight. Purify on PD-10 column	Eu labeling kit 1244-302 Wallac
β-Phycoerythrin–IgG	Derivatize both β-phycoerythrin and purified IgG with N-succinimidyl-3-(2-pyridyldithio)-propionate (SPDP). Cross-link using dithiothreitol. Purify on Sephacryl S300	9, 29

Table 7. Types of background fluorescence

Nature of background	τ (nsec)	Sources	Refs/comments
Rayleigh, Tyndall and large particle scattering	0	Particles and molecules	Increases with the addition of protein to solution [30, 31]
Raman scattering	0	Solvent molecules	Stokes' shift = 50 nm (λex = 350 nm) in distilled water or PBS [30, 31].
Sample fluorescence	2–10	Compounds in biological fluids	Stokes' Shift < 100 nm. The emission is most intense when λex < 350 nm and decreases as λex increases [1, 2]
Reagent fluorescence	2–10	Assay reagents	Antibodies etc. are fluorescent
Optics hardware and disposables			Some plastics show fluorescent emission

Fluorescent and Phosphorescent Labeled Assays

Chapter 8 CHEMILUMINESCENT AND BIOLUMINESCENT LABELED ASSAYS – S. Blincko

1 Introduction

The use of chemiluminescence for detection in immuno-assays is now routine. Chemiluminescent reactions are very sensitive to interference and so the analyte matrix is normally removed before end point determination.

The acridinium ester and enhanced luminescence systems are the two most commonly used strategies [1–3].

2 Chemiluminescence and bioluminescence

A compound that emits light following a chemical reaction is said to be chemiluminescent. Bioluminescence is a type of chemiluminescence where the reactants, catalysts, etc. are found in living organisms. In all cases the chemical/

peroxidase emits light over an extended time (> 30 min). e.g. peroxidase + luminol + *p*-iodophenol (chemical enhancer) + H_2O_2 at pH 8. The enhancer has the effect of prolonging the lifetime and enhancing the intensity of light production. This has enabled reliable application of enzyme assays with chemiluminescent substrates.

3 Luminometers and reagent addition

A range of luminometers is available. Those which gather light from all around the sample are the most sensitive. It is also possible to use a fluorimeter with the excitation source turned off to measure light intensity. For some applications where the greatest sensitivity is not required, light sensitive film may be employed [4].

biochemical reaction leads to the formation of electronic excited states which on decaying to the ground state emit photons. A typical chemiluminescent reaction, e.g. amino-butyl ethyl isoluminol (ABEI)+base (OH$^-$)+peroxidase (enzyme)+hydrogen peroxide (H$_2$O$_2$), gives a quick burst of light over about 7 sec. Acridinium ester + OH$^-$ + H$_2$O$_2$ gives a similar but shorter burst of light (over about 5 sec).

The light emission may be quantified in three ways (*Figure 1*):

1. peak light intensity (PLI);
2. decay part integration (DPI);
3. total light production (TLP).

The kinetics of these chemiluminescent reactions are dependent upon the rapid addition of reactants and their rate of mixing. Therefore, for fast reactions, rapid and precise reagent addition is necessary.

In contrast the enhanced chemiluminescence reaction with

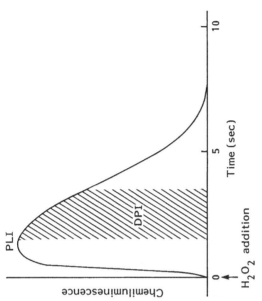

Figure 1. Chemiluminescence in terms of light intensity plotted against time.

Chemiluminescence and Bioluminescence

77

3.1 Reagent addition

Reagents for chemiluminescent reactions must be delivered in an accurate, precise and rapid way. For all methods clean instrumentation is vital. Many luminometers are equipped with special reagent injectors (e.g. dispensers for hydrogen peroxide to oxidize acridinium esters and isoluminol derivatives) [5].

Where plastic tubing is used to convey reagents it should be covered in tin foil or painted black. Samples may be held in test tubes or microtiter plates (clear or white).

4 Chemiluminescent and bioluminescent immunoassays

Table 1 lists the types of chemiluminescent and bioluminescent immunoassays in use.

5 Chemiluminescent and bioluminescent labels

Table 2 describes the labels used in chemiluminescent and bioluminescent immunoassays.

6 Enzyme-labeled chemiluminescent and bioluminescent systems

These are described in *Table 3*.

7 Preparation of labels

The chemistry involved is similar to that detailed for fluorescent labels (see Chapter 7).

8 Background and interference

Chemiluminescent reactions are very susceptible to factors that raise the background and interfere with the signal. For reliable running of chemiluminescent assays the greatest care must be taken to ensure the purity of reagents and the cleanliness of equipment (see *Table 4*).

Table 1. Chemiluminescent and bioluminescent immunoassays

Type of assay	Description	Refs
Chemiluminescence immunoassay	Antigen labeled with a chemiluminescent compound (e.g. isoluminol or an acridinium ester)	1, 6
Bioluminescence immunoassay	Antigen labeled with a bioluminescent compound	1, 6
Bioluminescence cofactor immunoassay	Antigen labeled with a cofactor that participates directly or indirectly with a chemiluminescent or bioluminescent reaction (e.g. adenosine triphosphate, ATP)	7, 8
Enzyme immunoassay with chemiluminescent or bioluminescent substrates	EIA and IEMA with a chemiluminescent enzyme substrate (e.g. HRP + luminol/H_2O_2/ enhancer). This method has found wide application	1, 2, 9
Immunochemiluminometric immunoassays	Antibody labeled with a chemiluminescent compound (e.g. acridinium ester)	1, 2, 5
Chemiluminescence enhancement (homogeneous)	Chemiluminescent emission is enhanced when antibody–antigen complex is formed. Also kinetics of light emission may be altered. Suffers interference from serum components	6, 10
Energy transfer immunoassay (homogeneous)	Antigen labeled with luminol derivative and antibody labeled with fluorescein isothiocyanate (FITC). Chemiluminescent reaction forms excited state of luminol which transfers its energy to FITC only when antigen–antibody complex is formed (i.e. when luminol and FITC are close) and so leads to emission at 520 nm. Ratio of 460 nm : 520 nm emission used to quantify assay so overcoming serum component interference	1, 11

Chemiluminescence and Bioluminescence

Table 2. Chemiluminescent and bioluminescent labels

Chemiluminescent compound	Reactants	λem (nm)	ϕ_{CL}	Comments
Luminol	OH⁻ H_2O_2 Microperoxidase	425–430	0.001 Unconjugated	Not preferred as a label for proteins/haptens due to drop in ϕ_{CL} on conjugation [1–3]
Isoluminol	OH⁻ H_2O_2 Microperoxidase	~430	0.0001 Unconjugated	Not preferred as a label for proteins/haptens unless substituted by alkyl groups (especially ABEI, see below) [1–3]
ABEI (aminobutyl ethyl isoluminol) A variety of labeling derivatives have been made	OH⁻ H_2O_2 Microperoxidase	~460	~0.0009 Unconjugated	Preferred over luminol as a label because ϕ_{CL} is not always markedly affected by conjugation
AHEI (aminohexyl ethylisoluminol)	H_2O_2 + microperoxidase + OH⁻	~460	~0.0009 Unconjugated	Used less frequently than ABEI [1]
ABENH (7-[N-4-amino butyl-N-ethylamino] naphthalene-1,2-amino-2,3-dihydrophthalazine-1,4-dione)	H_2O_2 + microperoxidase + OH⁻	>460		Also benzo [ghi] perylene derivative available [3]

		~460	~0.1	
Acridinium esters (derivatives with N-hydroxy succinimide active esters for labeling proteins and haptens)	OH^- H_2O_2 Pre-incubation at pH 5–7 followed by rapid jump in pH with H_2O_2 gives optimum light emission			Has found wide application [1–3] Simpler triggering of chemiluminescent reaction than for luminol series of compounds The chemiluminescent reaction involves detachment of the luminescing molecule, therefore protein/hapten conjugates have little effect on ϕ_{CL} However the ester linkage in original labels can be susceptible to hydrolysis and leads to a poorly chemiluminescent N-methyl acridylate. Newer acridinium esters, thioesters and sulphonyl carboxamides and phenanthridium esters are more stable [3]
Adamantane dioxetanes	Triggered by rapid heating			Derivatives must be thermally stable enough to avoid high background [2, 3, 12, 29]
Fluorescein	$Ca(OCl)_2$	525		Simple method [13]
Apoaequorin	Coelenterazine + Ca^{2+}	469		Recombinant apoaequorin is converted to aequorin which emits light [3, 12]

Chemiluminescence and Bioluminescence

81

Table 3. Enzyme-labeled chemiluminescent and bioluminescent systems

Enzyme or cofactor label	Reactants	Comment/refs
Horseradish peroxidase (HRP)	Luminol + H_2O_2 + OH^- + enhancer	Has found widespread application [1, 2, 9]. A nonseparation assay has been developed [14]. Numerous enhancers have been tested [9]
Manganese porphine derivative	Luminol + OH^- + O_2 (atmos) no H_2O_2 required	HRP mimetic. Light emission stable >20 min [12, 21]. Enhancers: Tween-20 and linoleic acid
Alkaline phosphatase	Firefly D-luciferin-O-phosphate + firefly luciferase + ATP + Mg^{2+}	The phosphate derivative will not react with luciferase until cleaved by alkaline phosphatase [15, 16]
Alkaline phosphatase	Adamantyl-1,2-dioxetane phenyl phosphate and derivatives	Most sensitive substrate for alkaline phosphatase [3, 12, 17, 18]. λem 477 nm lifetime > 1 h. Enhancers: polymers [19] or fluorescein + detergent (energy transfer) [20]
Luciferases (firefly, marine bacterial and recombinant)	Luciferin + ATP + Mg^{2+} + O_2	Quantum yields are high often > 0.3 [1, 3, 12]. Enhanced by nonionic surfactants. Natural luciferases lose activity on conjugation to proteins. Three methods have been devised to overcome this: 1. conjugation with biotin [22] 2. reversible conjugation [23] 3. recombinant luciferases [24]
Glucose-6-phosphate dehydrogenase	Isoluminol + multiple components	Complex series of reactions gives H_2O_2 which causes isoluminol + microperoxidase + OH^- to emit light [25]
Xanthine oxidase	Luminol + iron-EDTA complex	Very sensitive – lifetime of emission several days [26, 27]
β-Galactosidase	O-nitrophenyl galactoside + multiple components + marine luciferase	Complex series of reactions: the most sensitive bioluminescent method available [3, 28]
ATP (enzyme cofactor)	Firefly luciferase + luciferin + Mg^{2+}	7

| Nicotinamide adenine dinucleotide (NAD$^+$) (enzyme cofactor) | Ethanol + alcohol dehydrogenase + multiple components + marine luciferase | 8 |

Table 4. Background and interference

Sources of background and interference	Comments
Reagent bottles and injector tubing unprotected from light	All chemiluminescent reagents must be stored and transferred protected from light
Reagent impurities	1. Impurities may chemiluminesce under reaction conditions. All immunoassay procedures, reagents and equipment must be kept in a separate room to chemical synthesis or weighing of chemicals
	2. Impurities may interfere with the chemiluminescent reaction
Biological fluids	These are well known to affect chemiluminescent reactions in an unpredictable way. Most assays remove the biological matrix before end-point determination
Reaction background	Stability of the label or substrate is very important to diminish background

Chemiluminescence and Bioluminescence

Chapter 9 PRECIPITATION AND AGGLUTINATION METHODS – J. Little

1 Introduction

The reaction of antibody and antigen, the effective part of the humoral immune response, occurs in two stages *in vivo*. First, antigen is bound by antigen, forming a complex in dynamic equilibrium. Secondly, effector functions, such as complement activation, opsonization/macrophage binding and agglutination/precipitation. The latter occurs because antibody is divalent (has two binding sites) and naturally occurring antigens are usually multivalent. The precipitation/agglutination phenomenon is the basis of a variety of qualitative and quantitative *in vitro* laboratory techniques.

2 The precipitin test

The first quantitative immunoassay [1]. A liquid phase

3 Precipitation in gels

The quantitative aspects, efficiency and precision of the precipitin reaction are improved by the use of gel supports. There are two methods: diffusion of reagents and electrophoresis driven reagents.

Definitions of heterogeneity and antigenic identity obtained with these methods are serological and results are only comparable when the same reagents are employed.

3.1 General procedures

The methods are simple in principle but require particular operator skills to be successful. Details of reagents and apparatus specifically required for precipitin gel methods are given in *Table 1*; common methods are outlined in *Table 2*.

immunoprecipitation in which antigen, in various amounts, is added to a fixed quantity of antibody. A series of tubes are prepared containing antigen standards (typical range 10 μg to 1 mg) to which diluted antisera is added (e.g. 1:5–1:20 in PBS). The reaction is allowed to reach equilibrium and the mass of precipitates formed is determined. A biphasic relationship is obtained which can be used to:

1. calculate concentration of antibody in antiserum at the point of equivalence (no free antigen or antibody);
2. determine antigenic valency (when molecular mass of antigen and antibody is known).

The shape of the curve obtained varies with the nature of the antigen (valency; protein, polysaccharide, nucleic acid, etc.) and the properties of the antiserum (titer, avidity, etc.) which together produce immune complexes of different solubilities (dependent on overall molecular weight and features of the Fc portion of antibody).

Technical details are given in [2, 3].

3.2 Interpretation of precipitation patterns

The essential categories of techniques are given in *Table 3*. They serve as a basis of more sophisticated methods described in ref. 14. The appearance and meaning of typical precipitin patterns are shown in *Figure 1*.

4 Agglutination systems (visual end-point)

Distinct from precipitation, agglutination methodology employs particles, with linked Ab or Ag, to enhance the speed, sensitivity and visibility of the reaction. *Table 4* summarizes particles which have been used for immunoassay.

Traditional agglutination methodology with a visual end point allow semi-quantitative comparisons of antisera and determination of antigen concentrations. Antisera are diluted until they no longer give visible reactions with the same antigen: the end point. Antigen is assessed by its ability to inhibit an homologous agglutination system.

Precipitation and Agglutination Methods

1. SRID. Diameter of circles at equilibrium is proportional to Log (Ag concentration).

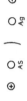

70   140   280   467   µg ml⁻¹

2. DID: basic patterns. Reaction of two antigens bearing combinations of epitopes X, Y and Z with AS. α−X = anti-X, α−Y = anti-Y, α−Z = anti-Z.

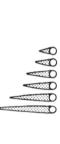

Shared epitope Y   X and Z not shared   Partial identity − shared Y, Z on one Ag only

N.B. Mixtures of antigens with (unlinked) epitopes may produce false results. The position of precipitin lines in relation to the wells is indicative of concentration (semi-quantitative).

3. IE. IE pattern for normal serum against anti-normal AS.

Albumin   Origin   IgC

⊕   ⊖

4. Cross-over electrophoresis

⊕   O   )   O   ⊖
    AS   Ag

N.B. IgG moves to cathode; electroendosmotic flow at pH 8.2.

5. Electroimmunoassay

AS in gel. Height of 'rocket' proportional to [Ag]

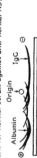

Reversed − Ag in gel

Figure 1. Appearance and interpretation of precipitin patterns. The simplest examples are shown. More complex procedures and 'false' results are fully discussed in ref. 14. SRID, single radial immunodiffusion; DID, double immunodiffusion; IE, immunoelectrophoresis.

4.1 Hemagglutination

The simplest example is agglutination of erythrocytes (RBC) by anti-erythrocyte serum. RBC can also be coated with Ag or Ab (*Table 5*). Coated RBC are used for passive hemagglutination (PH) [23] and reverse passive hemagglutination (RPH) [24], respectively.

In PH Ag-coated RBC are agglutinated by Ag specific antisera and in RPH Ab-coated RBC are agglutinated by the relevant Ag. As in all serological methods definitions are comparative. Reactions are typically carried out in V-bottomed microtiter plates: agglutination is evidenced by RBC not pelleting at the bottom of the well.

Presence of IgM in test sera is shown by β-mercaptoethanol (0.1 mM destroys IgM but not IgG binding). Control uncoated RBC are used to identify the presence of interference such as heterophilic antibodies (endogenous specimen Ab causing agglutination in the absence of Ag under test). If heterophilic Ab is present the specimen should be treated with PEG 6000 [29].

For sophisticated hemagglutination applications see [23, 24].

4.2 Latex agglutination

Latex particles are generally unsuitable for use in microtiter formats and are used extensively in light scattering systems (section 5). However, simple screening tests for rheumatoid factor, HBsAg and hCG (pregnancy) with coated latex particles have been widely used in a glass slide format [30]. Antiserum (in dilution PBS) is added to coated latex on the slide. Agglutination is visualized by illumination against a dark background.

5 Light scattering by particles

The formation of both immune complex and the agglutination of larger particles can be monitored by light scattering. Specialized instrumentation is required and rapid analyses of hundreds of samples daily with precision and sensitivity approaching labeled heterogeneous immunoassay is possible.

Precipitation and Agglutination Methods

Rayleigh scattering by small particles is given by:

$$i_\phi = I_0 \frac{8\Pi^4 N \alpha^2 (1 + \cos^2\phi)}{r^2 \lambda^4}$$

i_ϕ = scattered light at ϕ, I_0 = incident intensity, λ = wavelength, N = concentration of particles, α = molecular polarizability, and r = distance from particle to detector [31].

Theory predicts equal scattering forward and back. Immune complexes range in size from 50 to 100 nm and during complex formation Rayleigh scattering applies. In particle enhanced agglutination systems (e.g. latex particles of size around 500 nm) more complex scattering patterns result [32, 33]. Forward scattering occurs in all cases but optimum setting of the instrument (e.g. angle and wavelength) depends upon the size of particles, their density and the presence of other scattering species.

Light scattering methods are suitable for the assay of

5.2 Nephelometry

Nephelometry is an adaptation of the precipitin system. Immune complexes formed rapidly in suspension (no diffusion need occur) are illuminated in a photometer with monochromatic light [38]. Light scattering is measured by the intensity of light observed at angle ϕ to the incident beam. Instruments are designed to read forward scattering and ϕ is variable between $0°$ and $90°$. In practice nephelometry has comparable performance to turbidimetry but is less sensitive and precise, possibly because of increased specimen interference due to endogenous light scattering [39].

5.3 Particle counting (PC)

Using latex particles linked to Ab or Ag (see Chapter 4). The angle of light scattering depends upon the size of particles in suspension. By masking the detection optics a photometer can be set to quantify particles according to size, e.g. 600 nm latex particles; scattering by particles smaller than 600 nm

analytes in relatively high concentration (e.g. acute phase proteins, micro-organisms, drugs and hapten hormones such as cortisol and thyroxine).

5.1 Turbidimetry

The formation of complexes in suspension can be followed by the decrease in intensity of a beam of light by spectrophotometry. Loss of light is due to absorbtion, reflection and scatter and the signal obtained is dependent on wavelength, band width, amount of stray light, sample pathlength and the stability of light source and detector [34].

Turbidimetry can measure $20\,mg\,l^{-1}$–$5\,g\,l^{-1}$ but sample pretreatment (PEG 6000, protamine sulfate, dextran sulfate. $CaCl_2$ [35–37]) is essential for concentrations less than $50\,mg\,l^{-1}$.

and larger than 1200 nm is not counted [40, 41]. The technique is therefore used for counting unagglutinated particles. PC has greater sensitivity than turbidimetry or nephelometry because it does not require the formation of immune complexes large enough to scatter light.

5.4 Photon correlation spectroscopy (PCS)

A multichannel multiangular laser nephelometer with correlator can be used to determine the amount of *fluctuation* in light scattering due to Brownian motion [42]. Smaller particles move faster and therefore further in a given time than larger particles. a diffusion constant (for particles present) can be calculated by Fourier transform analysis and related to particle size. PCS requires sophisticated equipment and immunoassays, although more sensitive than turbidimetry or nephelometry, take longer to perform [43].

Precipitation and Agglutination Methods

Table 1. Reagents and equipment for precipitation in gel techniques

Item	Description and purpose	Recipes and details of use
Barbitone buffer	Suitable for general use; pH 8.2, ionic strength 0.08	12 g sodium 5'5 diethylbarbiturate dissolved in 150 ml dH_2O. 4.4 g 5'5 diethylbarbituric acid dissolved in 150 ml at 95°C. Mix and titrate to pH 8.2 with cNaOH. Add 0.2 g sodium azide and make up to 1l; store at 4°C.
Tris/barbitone buffer	Suitable in particular for electrophoretic procedures; pH 8.5, ionic strength 0.02, produces better separation, especially with high protein concentrations	4.48 g 5'5 diethylbarbituric acid, 8.86 g Tris, 0.2 g sodium azide, 0.4 g calcium lactate. Dissolve in dH_2O and make up to 1l; store at 4°C
Tris/Tricine	Barbitone is often difficult to obtain and is expensive (due to legal restrictions and drug control). A suitable general substitute for barbitone buffer which does not significantly alter precipitin patterns	4.52 g Tricine (N-tris(hydroxymethyl) glycine), 8.86 g Tris, 0.2 g sodium azide, 0.4 g calcium lactate. Dissolve in dH_2O and make up to 1l; store at 4°C
Agar and agarose	A mixture of polysaccharides, mainly of galactose and anhydrogalactose. Must be electrophoresis grade. Agar is recommended for general use and agarose (prepared by fractionation of agar) used preferentially for electrophoretic methods	(i) 1 or 2% agar or agarose in barbitone buffer, pH 8.2. Dissolve agar/agarose in 50 ml dH_2O with a boiling water bath/stirring hot plate, ensuring no lumps remain. Add 50 ml hot barbitone buffer & mix. Suitable for general immunodiffusion (add an equal volume of antibody or antigen solution in barbitone buffer to 2% gel). (ii) 1% agarose in tris/barbitone buffer, pH 8.6. Dissolve 1g agarose in 100 ml buffer with a boiling water bath/stirring hot plate. Store agar/agarose at 4°C for up to 2 months

Coomassie blue R 250 stain	For visualizing weak precipitin lines and preparing gels for photography	0.5% w/v in 9:9:2 ethanol:water:acetic acid. Dissolved by heating to 60°C, cooled and filtered. Stain for 5–10 min; destain 9:9:2 ethanol:water:acetic acid
Electrophoresis equipment	DC power supply up to 300 V/200 mA giving 10–15 V cm^{-1}	Use with Whatman No 1 filter paper wicks (soaked in buffer)
Gel punches	Metal tube/square-ended needles 2, 2.5, 3, 4 mm diameter, end sharpened, corresponding to 1–15 μl loading for gels 1.5 mm thick	Gel pierced; plug removed by suction/drawn-out Pasteur pipette. Single punches used with templates to arrange wells desired configurations, see Figure 1 for examples. Commercially available punches in various configurations are available
Slit former	For making rectangular wells particularly for electrophoretic separations	Placed on molten gel and removed after setting
Glass plates/plastic film	For supporting gels. 1 mm thick glass; common sizes (mm) 25 x 75, 50 x 50, 50 x 70, 100 x 100 and 11 x 205; select size for application required	To ensure adhesion pre-coat glass with a weak (0.5% in buffer) agar solution and allow to dry before casting or pouring gels. Plastic films have a hydrophilic side which adheres to gel
Levelling table	For preparing gels of even thickness	Table made horizontal just before use using integral spirit level
Miscellaneous	Sharp blades for cutting strips and slots, stirring hot plate for initial preparation of gel solutions, water bath for dissolving gel, equilibrating gel solutions and warming glass pipettes. etc.	

Precipitation and Agglutination Methods

Table 2. General procedures

Procedure	Method
Pouring gels	A dry pre-coated glass plate or plastic film support placed on a levelling table, may be insulated from the table with paper. Gel solution is dissolved in boiling water bath is cooled to 57°C, and antibody or antigen added as required. *N.B. denaturation of proteins increases with higher temperatures.* A portion of gel (volume determined from the area of support and a gel thickness of 1.5 mm) is placed in a suitable lipped test tube. The tube is dried and the warm gel quickly poured over the surface of the support (for small volumes, e.g. 2–4 ml, use a warmed wide bore glass pipette)
Casting gels	For absolutely even gel thickness use two glass plates, one uncoated, clamped together with a square U-shaped spacer of required thickness between. Once gel has set, remove uncoated plate by sliding counter to the spacer
Blotting/washing gels after immunodiffusion/electrophoresis	Nonprecipitated proteins are removed before staining. Draw water out of the gel by blotting with a contact filter paper, moistened with dH_2O, and layers of tissue paper, weighted down. After 15 min the blot is removed and the gel plate soaked in 0.9% saline for 15 min. The blotting and washing is repeated followed with a final wash in distilled water. Gels are dried with a warm air current
Staining of gels	Dried gels can be stained with Coomassie blue by immersion for 5–10 min. Destain by three washes of 10 min each and then dry the gel again. If destaining is too great repeat the staining procedure. The concentration of reagents in gel procedures makes this type of staining most suitable. If required for comparison with completed immunoelectrophoretic gels, first dimension electrophoresis gels can be fixed, with 1% picric acid in 16% acetic acid, dried and then stained
Viewing and recording of gels	Stain the precipitin lines (if necessary) and view on light box, gel side down. Dimension and position of precipitin lines are determined with an engineer's rule or micrometer scale with the use of dividers (if required). A photographic enlarger may be used too examine fine detail. Dried stained gels may be stored (particularly convenient if on plastic support) or photographed

Table 3. Summary of features and uses of basic gel techniques

Test name	Usage	Technical details	Ref.
Single radial immunodiffusion (SRID)	Quantitation of Ag	AS[a,b] incorporated with gel (at appropriate dilution). Ag (in dilution) added to circular wells cut in gel. Circular precipitin lines appear; at equilibrium diameter directly proportional to (log) antigen concentration	4, 5
Double immunodiffusion (DID)	Comparative test for antigenic identity–shared[b] determinants, partially shared determinants– or for comparison of antisera	Ag and AS added to circular wells cut in gel; both diffuse and form precipitin lines at point of equivalence. Usually AS or Ag under test put in multiple wells arranged around central well containing complimentary reagent; size, distance between and number of wells depend upon number and concentration of AS and Ag. Heterogeneous Ag and AS (mixed population specificities) will produce a number of lines	6, 7
Immunoelectrophoresis (IE)	Test of multiple antigenic identity in complex mixtures (e.g. serum). Able to show shared identity of physicochemically distinct molecules	Basic technique a combination of agar[d] electrophoresis and DID. Two stages: Ag mixture separated linearly by electrophoresis; AS added in slot cut into the gel parallel to direction of separation and Ag diffusing form multiple precipitin lines	8, 9
Cross-over electrophoresis	Rapid analysis of multiple samples for specific detection of Ag	Electrophoretically driven DID at pH 8.2. Two circular wells cut in agar gel slab, AS put in well nearest anode, Ag in well nearest cathode. Ab (IgG, no	10

continued

Precipitation and Agglutination Methods

Immunoassays

Table 3. Summary of features and uses of basic gel techniques, *continued*

Test name	Usage	Technical details	Ref.
		charge) migrate towards cathode due to electoendosmotic flow, Ag (negative charge) to anode; precipitin lines form at equivalence. Method uses less reagent than DID as Ab and Ag driven together rather than diffusing radially	
Electroimmunoassay or 'Rocket' electrophoresis	Rapid and accurate identification and quantitation of Ag, sensitivity 1 µg ml^{-1}. Elucidation of partial antigenic identity	Electrophoresis of antigen, from a point source, in agarose gel containing the corresponding antibody. Circular wells cut in gel, most Ag migrate towards the anode; agarose used to reduce electroendosmosis	11, 12
Crossed immunoelectrophoresis	Antigen subpopulation quantitation in heterogeneous populations, more rapid than IE. Comparison of antisera	A hybrid of IE and electroimmunoassay. After separation of antigens by agar electrophoresis they are driven into an antibody containing gel by an electric field at right angles to the original. A strip is cut from the first electrophoretic slab which is placed in an accurately cut slot in the Ab gel. Precipitin line(s) are formed; the area enclosed by the line and the gel strip is proportional to the total mass of antigen	13

[a]AS = antiserum. Purified or partially purified Ab may be substituted (Chapter 2).

[b]In reverse SRID Ag incorporated with gel.

[c]Serologically defined with reference to a particular antiserum.

[d]At pH 8.2 β_2- and γ-globulins migrate to cathode due to electroendosmosis effect. Agarose may be used to reduce the effect.

Table 4. Particles for immunoassay systems

Particle	Mode of detection	Usage	Ref.
Bacteria	Visual	Semi-quantitative assay of Ab and Ag.	15
Erythrocytes	Visual	Blood grouping. Quantitative assays	16
Metal sols Au, Ag, AgI BaSO$_4$	Light scattering	Quantitative assay of Ag & Ab	17, 18
Latex	Visual, light scattering	Screening tests for Ag & Ab, eg autoantibody on slide format (particle size > 500 nm) Quantitative assays by light scattering	19–22

Table 5. Linkage of Ab and Ag to erythrocytes

Assay type	Method	Ref.
RPH	Pretreat with trypsin to reduce surface charge (zeta potential). Chromic chloride in piperazine or imidazole buffer, pH 6.5	25
RPH	Glutaraldehyde	26
PH, polysaccharide Ag	Spontaneous coupling to cell surface	27
PH, protein Ag	Cells treated with tannic acid (2.5% in PBS, pH 7.4) and formalin (4% in borate/succinate 150 mM, pH 7.5); control cells receive no Ag	28

Precipitation and Agglutination Methods

95

Chapter 10 DRY SURFACE IMMUNOASSAYS AND IMMUNOSENSORS –
R. Edwards

1 Introduction

The development of dry surface immunoassays and immunosensors has been motivated by the obvious convenience and success of certain dip-stick tests and dry-reagent clinical assays, such as that for measuring glucose. Immunosensors can be viewed as logical but specialized developments of more basic sensor technology. The advantages of dry surface (film) immunoassays and immunosensors are:

1. simple to use by inexperienced or untrained operators;
2. primarily portable, to be used independently of specialist facilities, i.e. laboratories;
3. measurement independent of sample volume or matrix;
4. potentially disposable and inexpensive devices;
5. re-usable or continuous measurement formats;

different materials (e.g. paper, gelatin, agarose, methylcellulose, etc.) Detection in automated analyzers usually depends upon reflective photometry using enzyme reactions generating colored products or front-surface fluorimetry using fluorophores (also sometimes as products from enzyme reactions).

Table 1 lists a variety of systems illustrating the range of possible formats.

Other useful features of dry surface devices include:

1. grooved surfaces to enable sample to spread evenly over surface of device;
2. use of gelatin layer to prevent penetration of high molecular proteins and thus remove potential interference in sample;

6. rapid;
7. capable of measuring multiple analytes.

In general, very simple devices developed to exploit dry surface immunoassays lack sensitivity and as such have limited application to analytes present in relatively high concentrations (e.g. human chorionic gonodotrophin (HCG) in pregnancy tests). Sensitivity can certainly be extended when they are used in connection with sophisticated automated analyzers, or as predicted for the multianalyte 'microspot immunoassay' [1].

2 Dry surface systems

In these devices the antibody reagent or reagents are immobilized in various ways on permeable or porous membranes. In some cases the other reagents are applied as liquids and in others they are dried on or in the membrane. The simplest type are single element units, whilst others have multi-layered membranes, often using

3. use of wheatgerm agglutinin or antiserum to human erythrocytes to retard capillary migration of red blood cells, enabling use of whole blood as sample;
4. use of absorptive layer (e.g. containing iron oxide to limit 'background' detection);
5. use of reflective layers (e.g. containing TiO_2 or $BaSO_4$ to enhance reflection to photometer).

3 Immunosensors

Immunosensors, in terms of practical application, are still at an early stage of development. Although they are predicted to manifest all aspects of an ideal detector or sensor, practical constraints and sensitivities remain to be elucidated.

Table 2 lists the principal technologies with potential for immunosensors.

The practicality of immunosensors using surface plasmon resonance is demonstrated by the BIAcore™ developed by

Dry Surface Immunoassays and Immunosensors

Pharmacia. In this instrument samples are transported to the sensor chip surface in a flow cell (integrated fluidic cartridge). Antibodies are immobilized on a flexible matrix of carboxymethylated dextran. The BIAcore™ enables real-time analysis of every stage of complex interactions as well as rapid and automated measurement of an analyte.

Undoubtedly the most exciting aspect of immunosensor developments is the potential for a miniaturized array of tests for a variety of analytes on microdots. A system based on dual label laser scanning confocal fluorescence micro-scopic measurements, ratiometric' microspot immunoassays, under commercial development by Boehringer, promises the measurement of many different analytes within an area barely visible to the naked eye [1].

Table 1. Specific examples of dry surface immunoassays

Antibody format	Other reagents	Measurement
Immobilized on nylon membrane	Applied as liquids pulled through porous polythylene disc on to cellulose acetate absorbent	Color by comparison with control (visual) (e.g. Hybritech Icon® pregnancy test)
Immobilized antibody immune complex on glass fiber membrane	Reaction carried out on analyzer with fluid reagent dispensers to facilitate radial partition immunoassay	Front-surface fluorimetry (enzyme reaction) (e.g. Baxter Stratus®)
Immobilized on paper chromatographic strip	Dipped into fluid reagents to facilitate capillary migration	Height of colored bar (visual) (e.g. Syva AccuLevel®)
Impregnated cellulose paper	Sequential drying of all other reagents including enzyme substrate	Intensity of color by reflectance photometry (e.g. Miles ARIS™)
Immobilized on porous membrane	All reagents including colored latex particles on porous membrane, also use of sampling wick	Position of colored band (visual) (e.g. Unipath Clearblue® pregnancy test)

99   *Dry Surface Immunoassays and Immunosensors*

Table 2. Principal technologies with potential for immunosensors

Type of immunosensor	Potential use	Ref.
Electrochemical immunosensors		
Potentiometric	Measurement of membrane or electrode potential after reaching equilibrium at sensor interface	2, 3
Amperometric	Measurement of current; an externally applied potential drives electrode reaction	2, 3
Potentiometric/amperometric with enzyme labels	Either type of electrochemical immunosensor can be used in conjunction with enzyme label to generate electroactive product	2, 3
Piezoelectric immunosensors		
Piezoelectric transducers	Measurement of changes in vibrational resonant frequency of piezoelectric quartz oscillators	3
Optical (evanescent wave) immunosensors		
Fluorescent evanescent-wave	Measurement of fluorescence arising from excitation of bound fraction by evanescent wave	4
Surface plasma resonance	Change of angle at which surface plasma resonance occurs	4

Chapter 11 DATA PROCESSING – I. Howes

1 Introduction

Any processing of complex data, such as: curve fitting to the dose–response coordinates for a number of replicated standards or calibration curve; precision profiling; interpolation of unknown values; statistical calculation of quality control parameters, etc. is best achieved using one of several computer programs (e.g. Multicalc or Ria-aid).

Laboratory analysts are usually ill-equipped to evaluate the data by eye for subtleties of nonlinearity, significant variation from a mean, heteroscedasticity, etc. Manual methods may miss important and essential information. Low cost, ready availability and demonstrably superior performance ensure the expedient and universal use of microprocessor-based data processing.

In this chapter data processing for quantitative immunoassays is considered to consist of the following steps:

1. calculation of mean response from replicates;
2. construction of the calibration curve;
3. assessment of quality of fit of the calibration curve;
4. determination of unknown concentration from the mean response;
5. construction of the precision profile;
6. estimation of sensitivity;
7. quality control.

2 Calculation of mean response from replicates

For a series of n replicate responses y_i, the mean response is given by:

$$\bar{y} = \frac{\sum\limits_{y=i}^{y=n} y_i}{n}$$

where:

$\bar{y}$ = mean response; y_i = individual response; n = number of replicates.

The standard deviation SD is given by:

$$SD = \sqrt{\frac{\sum\limits_{i=1}^{i=n} (\bar{y} - y_i)^2}{(n-1)}}$$

where:

SD = standard deviation; y_i = individual response; $\bar{y}$ = mean response; n = number of replicates.

An alternative equation for the standard deviation in which prior knowledge of the mean is not required is:

Adjacent response–concentration coordinates may be joined with straight lines in the technique of linear interpolation.

Manual plotting after transformation of the raw data

A series of reciprocal plots given below may linearize raw data:

y-axis	x-axis
$1/B$	linear dose
T/B	linear dose
B_0/B	linear dose
F/B	linear dose

where B = bound response (tracer bound by antibody); T = total response (tracer added to assay); B_0 = zero bound response (tracer bound by antibody in the absence of analyte); F = free response (tracer not bound by antibody).

The LOGIT transform may also linearize raw data. This is given by:

$$\text{Logit } Y = \log_e \left(\frac{y}{100-y}\right)$$

where the most commonly used response y is given by

$$y = \frac{\text{bound response} - (\text{nonspecific response})}{(\text{maximum bound response}) - (\text{nonspecific response})}$$

The percent coefficient of variation (%CV) is given by:

$$SD = \sqrt{\frac{\sum\limits_{i=1}^{i=n}(y_i^2) - \frac{\left(\sum\limits_{i=1}^{i=n}y_i\right)^2}{n}}{n-1}}$$

$$\%CV = \left(\frac{SD}{\text{mean}}\right) \times 100.$$

3 Construction of the calibration curve

The response–concentration coordinates obtained for each of the calibrators (known analyte concentration) require linking to form a monotonic, smooth and continuous curve [1–3].

3.1 Manual methods

Direct manual plotting

The raw data is plotted on graph paper and the resulting curve is drawn with a 'flexicurve', or other curve drawing aid.

3.2 Computer methods – mathematical modelling

Both radioimmunoassay (RIA) response curves and to a greater extent immunometric response curves (IRMA) suffer from nonuniformity of variance of the response variable with analyte concentration, this is known as heteroscedacity [4]. This heteroscedacity is clearly visible in the error profile (also known as response error relationship, RER). A weighting function should be used to accommodate this nonuniformity of variance. It is common to use $(1/SD^2)$ as a weighting factor for each calibrator such that replicates with larger variances will have less influence over the final position of the curve than those with smaller variances.

Point to point methods

Linear interpolation. Adjacent response–concentration co-ordinates are linked with straight lines.

Data Processing

Immunoassays

The equation of the straight line is

$$y = a + bx$$

where a = intercept on y-axis; b = gradient (slope) of the line.

Spline interpolation. Adjacent response–concentration coordinates are linked with section of polynomial functions.

The polynomial functions have equations

$$y = a + bx + cx^2 + dx^3$$

where y = response; a, b, c and d are parameters specific to each section of curve; x = concentration of calibrator.

Smoothed spline interpolation. Mathematical smoothing which prevents changes in the sign of the gradient between adjacent response–concentration coordinates is applied to the curve constructed with splines. The smoothing techniques are analogous to the way in which the straight line can be forced through the origin.

$$RSS = \sum_{i=1}^{i=n} (\hat{y}_i - \bar{y}_i)^2$$

where $\hat{y}$ = modeled response; $\bar{y}$ = mean response.

Linear regression. Regression may be applied to data which has been linearized by a transformation.

$$\vec{y} = a + bx$$

where $\vec{y}$ = transformed response, e.g. T/B etc.; a = intercept on y-axis; b = gradient (slope) of the line); x = calibrator concentration.

The application of least squares analysis to a straight line is referred to as linear regression.

Polynomial functions

$$y = a + bx + cx^2 + dx^3 + ex^4$$

where y = response; a, b, c, d, e are parameters specific to each curve; x = calibrator concentration. The highest power of x will define the nomenclature of the polynomial function (i.e. x^2 defines a quadratic, x^3 defines a cubic, and x^4 defines a quartic).

Logistic equations. The four parameter logistic equation (see *Figure 1*) [5] is defined by

$$y = \frac{(a - d)}{1 + (\frac{x}{c})^b} + d$$

where y = response; a = response at high asymptote (zero dose (RIA) or high dose (IRMA)); b = Slope factor; c = ED$_{50}$, the concentration corresponding to 50% specific binding; d = response at low asymptote (high dose (RIA) or zero dose (IRMA)); x = calibrator concentration.

The five parameter logistic equation is defined by

$$y = \frac{(a - d)}{[1 + (\frac{x}{c})^b]m} + d$$

To describe this formally one needs to adopt the 'functional' notation.

The cubic spline is defined by

$$F_1(x) = a_1 + b_1 x + c_1 x^2 + d_1 x^3$$

over the interval x_1, x_{1+1}

Imposing the condition that $F_1(x) = y_1$ ensures that the curve passes through all the calibration points, The further conditions $F'_1(x_1) = F'_{1-1}(x_1)$ and $F''_1(x_1) = F''_{1-1}(x_1)$ ensure that the shapes and curvatures of the curves are equal at each point.

Regression methods

Regression methods consider the vertical distance between the modeled and observed responses (the residuals).

$$\text{Residual} = (\hat{y}_i - \bar{y}_i)$$

The least squares method minimizes the sum of the squares of the differences between the modeled and observed response (the residual sum of squares, RSS).

Data Processing

where y = response; a = response at high asymptote (zero dose (RIA) or high dose (IRMA)); b = slope factor; c = ED$_{50}$, the concentration corresponding to 50% specific binding; d = response at low asymptote (high dose (RIA) or zero dose (IRMA)); x = calibrator concentration; m = asymmetry factor.

Notably in IRMA type assays the calibration curve lacks symmetry, the inclusion of the fifth parameter a so called asymmetry factor, permits modification of the four parameter logistic equation to accommodate this situation.

Law of mass action based models. The single binding site equation based on the law of mass action proposed by Ekins and Newman [6] has the form:

$$[(D + p^* + c) \cdot b + q] \cdot R^2 + [c \cdot (b+1) + q - p^* - D] \cdot R + c = 0$$

where R = free/bound ratio; p^* = tracer concentration; D = analyte dose; q = antibody concentration; c = 1/affinity constant; b = nonspecific binding.

The law of mass action equation devised by Wilkins [8] has the form:

$$Y = \frac{2P(1-B)}{K + P + A + X + [(K - P + A + X) + 4KP]^{\frac{1}{2}}} + B$$

where Y = response (antibody bound counts/total counts); K = equilibrium dissociation constant; P = antibody concentration; A = labeled antigen concentration; B = fraction of counts due to nonspecific-binding; X = analyte dose.

4 Assessment of quality of fit of the calibration curve

Examine the size of the sum of residuals, this is directly proportional to the quality of fit. Examine the individual residuals, points with high residuals may be 'outliers', points which do not fit the model and may require removal [9]. Calculate the predicted concentration of the calibrators from the response as if they were unknowns. Examine these values

There are six major assumptions in the model:

1. antigen and antibody are both monovalent;
2. the reaction is at equilibrium;
3. the equilibrium constants of labeled and unlabeled antigens are identical;
4. bound and free fraction are separated perfectly;
5. there are no cross-reacting species present;
6. the antibodies form a single population.

The multi-binding site model based on the law of mass action proposed by Ekins and co-workers [7] has the form:

$$R_{b/f} = \sum_{i=1}^{n} \frac{q_i}{\dfrac{p}{1 + R_{b/f}} + \dfrac{1}{K_i}}$$

where $R_{b/f}$ = bound response/free response; q_i = concentration of the reaction sites; p = analyte concentration (labeled and unlabeled); K_i = equilibrium constant at i^{th} reaction site.

for trends. Statistical variance ratio test: calculate the model variance, the deviation from the model averaged over all doses (s1). Calculate the replicate variance, the scatter of the replicate calibrators about their respective means averaged over all doses (s2). Form the variance ratio s1/s2, this is directly proportional to the quality of fit.

5 Determination of unknown concentrations from the mean response

Since the unknown mean response will fall between two calibrator responses for which the analyte concentration is known, the unknown concentration may be interpolated. For manual methods, the unknown concentration is read from the intersection of the line joining the response to the curve directly (see Figure 2).

For computer methods, since the mathematical function for the calibration curve is defined, the concentration corresponding to a response can be obtained by changing the

Data Processing

subject of the equation from response to concentration. Using the 'functional notation'

$$Resp = F(Conc)$$

becomes

$$Conc = F(Resp)$$

6 Construction of the precision profile

The sum of errors associated with measured responses are a function of concentration. This is illustrated by expressing the response error as an equivalent concentration error and plotting against concentration [10].

6.1 Intra-assay intra-sample precision profile using calibrators and samples

Without binning

1. Calculate the mean response ($\bar{y}$) and standard deviation in response (SD) for each set of replicates.

9. To obtain a precision profile in terms of SD, plot the concentration error against concentration.

10. To obtain a precision profile in terms of % coefficient of variation (%CV) divide the concentration error by the concentration at which it occurs and multiply the result by 100, this is the %CV and should be plotted against the concentration.

This approach requires a large number of sample to be assayed in replicate. Once obtained the profile is stable and can be used to monitor modifications in the assay.

With binning

1. Calculate the mean response ($\bar{y}$) and standard deviation in response (SD) for each set of replicates.

2. Plot the mean response against concentration for the calibrators. This is the calibration curve.

3. Square the standard deviation in response for each set of replicates to obtain the variance in response.

4. Divide the concentration range of the assay into 5–10 'bins' (smaller concentration ranges). Sum the variances

2. Plot the mean response against concentration for each of the calibrators. This is the calibration curve.
3. Plot the standard deviation in response against response. This is the response error relationship (RER) or error profile.
4. Use linear regression to fit a straight line to the error profile.
5. Select 5–10 points across the concentration range of the assay from which the precision profile will be calculated. Use the calibration curve to calculate the response at these concentrations.
6. Use the error profile to calculate the error (SD) in response at these levels.
7. Calculate the gradient of the calibration curve at each of the above concentration levels.
8. Use the gradient of the calibration curve to transform the response errors at each level to concentration errors.

$$\text{Error of concentration} = \frac{\text{SD of response}}{\text{Slope of response curve at this point}}$$

of response in each 'bin' and average. The 'bin' will be represented by the single average variance value.
5. Plot the average 'bin' variance against the average 'bin' concentration. This is the response error relationship (RER) error profile.
6. Use least squares regression to fit one of two models to data variance $= a + b\bar{y} + c\bar{y}^2$ or variance $= a(\bar{y})^b$.
7. Calculate the modeled variance for each bin from the curve in (6) above, calculate the square root of the variance to obtain the standard deviation (SD).
8. Calculate the gradient of the calibration curve at concentration levels corresponding to each mean 'bin' concentration.
9. Use the gradient of the calibration curve to transform the SD in response for each 'bin' to concentration errors.

$$\text{Error of concentration} = \frac{\text{SD of response}}{\text{Slope of response curve at this point}}$$

10. To obtain a precision profile in terms of SD plot the concentration error against concentration.

Data Processing

11. To obtain a precision profile in terms of % coefficient of variation (%CV) divide this concentration error by the average concentration value of the 'bin' and multiply the result by 100 to obtain %CV. Plot %CV against concentration.

This approach requires a large number of replicates at several analyte levels within the assay.

6.2 Intra-sample inter-assay precision profiles

These precision profiles are usually constructed by selecting a series of quality control samples spanning the entire analyte concentration range of interest and including them in several successive assay runs. This yields an estimate of the inter standard deviation.

The total error associated with a response is the sum of the experimental error and the measuring error:

$$SD^2_{total} = SD^2_{exp} + SD^2_{count}$$

Precision profiles are often presented where the measuring

7 Estimation of sensitivity

The sensitivity of an assay (the lowest concentration of analyte which can be distinguished from zero) is a function of the slope of the calibration curve and the precision at each dose [11]. The minimal detectable concentration (MDC) is calculated from the mean zero response plus a multiple of standard deviations of the response at this level estimated from the error profile See *Figure 3*. Precision profiles have been used directly, sensitivity being defined as the concentration corresponding to a CV of 22%.

Many simultaneous assays of the IRMA type which measure analytes over a wide concentration range have biphasic response curves. The concept of a maximum secure concentration has been proposed for such assays (see *Figure 4*).

8. Quality control

8.1 Estimation of internal quality control parameters

Parameters available from the calibrators

Maximum response (B_{max}). In 'RIA type assays' this will be

error is separated from the experimental (nonmeasuring error). In the case of radiolabeled immunoassays, this separation is relatively easy since the counting error is the square root of the counts accumulated.

Thus,
$$SD^2_{exp} = SD^2_{total} - SD^2_{count}$$

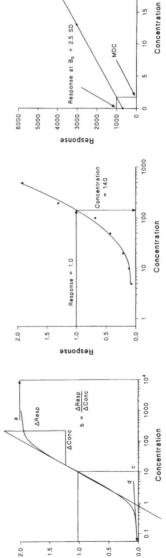

Figure 1. A four parameter logistic equation curve defining the four parameters and their influence on the slope of the curve.

Figure 2. Interpolation – the concentration is read from the intersection of the response ordinate with the calibration curve.

the binding in the absence of the analyte (B_0). In 'IRMA type assays' this will be the binding of the most concentrated calibrator.

Minimum response (B_{min}). In 'RIA type assays' this will be the nonspecific binding (NSB). In 'IRMA type assays' this

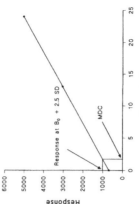

Figure 3. Minimal detectable concentration (MDC) as defined by 2.5 SD response from zero interpolated from the standard curve.

Immunoassays

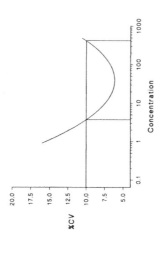

Figure 4. Maximum secure concentration (MSC) as defined by the concentration corresponding to the response to below which the highest expected concentration will not reduce the response.

will be the nonspecific binding associated with the zero analyte calibrator.

Parameters available from the calibration curve

1. ED_{50}, the concentration corresponding to a response

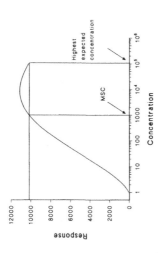

Figure 5. The precision profile and working range as defined by the appropriate %CV.

correspond to normal and abnormal levels of the analyte being measured. Bias is a measure of how far the assay value is from the 'true' value; precision is a measure of the reproducibility of the assay results (see *Figure 6*).

which is 50% of the specific binding. Numerically this is $(B_{max} - B_{min})/2 + NSB$.

2. ED_{20}, the concentration corresponding to a response which is 20% of the specific binding: numerically $(B_{max} - B_{min})/5 + NSB$.

3. ED_{80}, the concentration corresponding to a response which is 80% of the specific binding: numerically $(B_{max} - B_{min})/0.8 + NSB$.

4. The slope of the linear portion of the calibration curve.

Parameters available from the precision profile

The 'working range' can be identified from the precision profile as the range over which the assay has acceptable precision. 10% is frequently chosen to define the working range of the assay.

Minimum detectable concentration has been estimated from the precision profile (see *Figure 5*).

Parameters available from quality control pools

The concentration of the quality control pools should

113

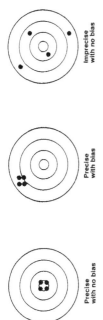

Figure 6. Precision and bias.

Shewhart/Levey Jennings plot. On a Shewhart/Levey Jennings plot, the mean value of the quantity being monitored is represented by a central axis [12]. This axis is flanked on either side by a set of warning limits placed at $+/- 2$ SD, and then by a set of action limits placed at $+/- 3$ SD. Sequential results are plotted progressing from left to right across the control chart (*Figure 7*). When a point strays outside the limits, the assay is said to be out of control.

CUSUM plots. On a cumulative sum CUSUM plot [13], the target mean is represented by a central axis, the cumulative

Data Processing

Immunoassays

for one unit on the vertical CUSUM axis is defined as *b*. The scaling factor *w* is defined by the ratio *b/a*. This should be approximately 2 SD.

3. Determine the performance characteristics of the chart. Select a value for the acceptance criterion Δ, this is the tolerance level statistic which is usually +/− 2 SD from the mean. Define the average run length for an out of control system L_2. This is the average number of points which will be plotted on the chart if there is a shift of the true mean away from the target mean, it is generally in the region of five and should be kept as small as possible.

4. Construct the V mask (see *Figures 8* and *9*). The nomogram relating Δ, L_1 and L_2 is required. Calculate the value Δ/2 SD and locate this on scale 1. On scale 2 locate the value for L_2. Use a straight edge to read the intersections of the line joining these two points with scales 3 and 4. The value obtained from scale 3 is *h*/SD, multiply this by SD to obtain the value for *h*. The lead distance *d* for the V mask is then calculated from the equation $d = (2wh)/\Delta$. The half angle of the vertex of the V mask is calculated from $\theta = \tan^{-1}(h/d)$. The value of

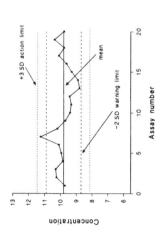

Figure 7. Shewhart/Levey Jennings control chart. A single control will stray outside the ^{1}2SD limits for one assay in 20.

difference of successive assays from the target mean is represented by the vertical axis. Values of the CUSUM are plotted sequentially from left to right on the chart.

$$\text{CUSUM} = \sum_{i=1}^{i=n} (\bar{x} - x_i)$$

A scaling factor is required for the axes. In the absence of any bias, the values for the CUSUM should fluctuate around zero. When a change in the target mean ($\bar{x}$) occurs there is a marked change in profile both in direction and magnitude of the slope.

A test is performed on each new measurement to see if the method detects a shift away from the target mean. A 'V' shaped mask (V mask) is held over the point to be tested. The central axis of the V mask must be parallel to the horizontal axis of the CUSUM plot, and the point being tested is located at a distance d (the lead distance away from the vertex of the V mask). If any of the points on the chart fall outside the limbs of the V mask, the assay is declared to be out of control with respect to the quality control parameter being monitored.

CUSUM chart plotting.

1. Calculate the target mean ($\bar{x}$) and standard deviation (SD) from a large number of assays.
2. Calculate the appropriate scale for the chart. The length representing one unit on the horizontal axis (the distance between successive assays) is defined as a. The distance

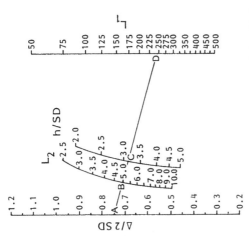

Figure 8. V mask nomogram showing the relationship between L_1, L_2 and Δ. Redrawn from ref. 13 by permission of the Journal of Endocrinology Ltd.

Data Processing

115

material when the last four values of the same control material exceed the same, i.e. mean + 1 SD or mean − 1 SD limit. The rule is violated across control materials when the last four consecutive values for different control levels exceed the same mean + 1 SD or mean − 1 SD limit.

6. Rule 10_x: this rule is applied both within and across control materials. The rule is violated across control materials when the last 10 consecutive control values regardless of control level, are on the same side of the mean. The rule is violated within the control material when the last 10 values for the same control level are all on the same side of the mean. This rule may be modified to nine values when running three control levels or eight values when running four control levels.

Application of the 1_{2s} rule alone (failure to include valid points between mean +/−2 SD and mean +/−3 SD) would falsely reject 5% of analytical runs using one level of control, 10% of analytical runs using two levels of control, and 14% of analytical runs using three levels of control.

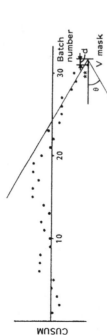

Figure 9. V mask and CUSUM. The V mask placed over each point will declare the assay out of control when one of the points is outside the limits of the mask. d = lead distance; θ = half angle; ** = out of control.

L_1 on the fourth scale is the average run length for an assay in control. This is the average number of points which will be plotted in a system (with no shift from the target mean) before random error will falsely cause the system to be declared out of control. This should be kept as high as possible.

Multi rule Shewhart quality control scheme. A number of rules have been proposed for quality control [14]. The six commonly used rules are as follows.

1. Rule 1_{2s}: this rule is violated when one measurement exceeds the mean $+/- 2$ SD.

2. Rule 1_{3s}: this rule is violated when one value exceeds the mean $+/- 3$ SD. The rule is applied within run only.

3. Rule 2_{2s} or (2 out of 3_{2s}): this rule is violated within the run when two consecutive control values (or two of three control values when three levels are being run) exceed the same limit, i.e. mean $+ 2$ SD or mean $- 2$ SD. The rule is violated across runs when the previous value for a particular control exceeds the same, i.e. mean $+ 2$ SD or mean $- 2$ SD limit.

4. Rule R_{4s}: this rule is applied within run only. It is violated when the difference between two consecutive control values (or two of three control values when three levels are being run) exceeds 4 SD.

5. Rule 4_{1s}: this rule is applied both within and across the control materials. The rule is violated within the control

The following rule combinations are used dependent upon the number of control levels used.

1. One control level per assay ($1_{2s}/4_{1s}$).
2. Two control levels per assay ($1_{3s}/2_{2s}/R_{4s}/4_{1s}/10_{\bar{x}}$).
3. Three control levels per assay ($1_{3s}/2$ of $3_{2s}/R_{4s}/9_{\bar{x}}$).
4. Four control levels per assay ($1_{3s}/2_{2s}/R_{4s}/4_{1s}/8_{\bar{x}}$).

Interpretation of the rules requires experience. Appropriate action will depend upon the specific circumstances.

Combined Shewhart and CUSUM chart. Quality control data plotted on a Shewhart chart is screened prior to the CUSUM being plotted. The CUSUM technique is modified to desensitize it.

1. Data points are allowed within the range target mean $+/-0.5$ SD without accumulating a CUSUM value.

2. Whenever the current Shewhart point is on the opposite side of the mean from the previous data point the CUSUM chart is zeroed.

117

Data Processing

Parameters available from samples

Assay means. The mean of assay results provides a useful quality control (QC) parameter. It is usually stable over several assays and a change may indicate deterioration of assay reagents. The mean may be trimmed for certain analytes.

Drift controls. Drift, the time related bias can be assessed by including repeated sets of quality control samples within the assay.

1. Use values of *t* (from Student's *t*-test tables) and precision data from the precision profile at the level of the QC to assess the significance any difference.

2. **Rank Sum test.** Each level of quality control is assigned a value according to its position in the rank, these values are summed across the assay and tables consulted to assess the significance of the range.

3. **Youden analysis.** When the quality control pool are run at the beginning and end of the assay, the values can be

of values, but are not necessarily outliers and are therefore retrieved for the later calculation of individual bias and variability of bias. The dispersion of the raw results cannot be calculated from the SD of the log data. To obtain a measure of this dispersion the GCV is calculated. Results reported as 'greater than' or 'less than' are excluded from the calculation.

Bias and its variability

By subtracting the log of the ALTM from the log of the laboratory's result on each usable sample, the bias is calculated. The biases are ranked and trimmed as for results, the mean and standard deviation are calculated. The bias is the mean log bias expressed as a percentage difference from 100. The variability of the bias is the GCV of the log bias values.

Youden plot for comparison of external QCs

The Youden technique requires the distribution and assay of matched pairs of quality control samples in which the concentration of the analyte is the same. The plot is constructed as follows; each laboratory (result) is represented by a single point the x-ordinate of which represents the value obtained for the first of the pair of samples and the y-ordinate is the second value.

Bias will affect both measurements equally and will push points on the Youden plot along the 45° line. Random errors will push points away from the 45° line (see Figure 10).

On the Youden plot in Figure 10 point A represents an assay with good accuracy that is precise and shows little bias, B an assay with positive bias and good precision, C an assay with negative bias and good precision, and the points D represent poor precision.

9 Guidelines for data processing (Special Report 1985)

The following guidelines were published in *Clinical Data Processing*

compared on a similar plot to the Youden plot used for comparison of external quality controls.

8.2 External quality assessment schemes (proficiency testing)

External quality control provides a means for independent assessment of laboratory performance. Sets of control samples are distributed to all laboratories participating in the scheme on a regular basis. No target values are provided with the samples and they are handled in the same way as patient samples. Results are returned to the schemes where they are collated and analysed. All participants are then provided with a report of the results.

Statistical calculations

All laboratory trimmed mean (ALTM) and geometric coefficient of variation (GCV). The results on each sample are transformed into their natural logarithms and ranked. The lowest and highest 5% of the results (rounded up to the nearest even number) are trimmed off. The excluded results play no part in the calculations of mean value and dispersion

Chemistry in 1985 [15]. The two modeled variables of the calibration curve are raw response (e.g. counts, and analyte concentration). The models to fit the calibration curves need flexibility of shape and position to suit the requirements of standard assay techniques. The models must also be monotonic in form and have restraint from making detours for outlying points. The four parameter logistic model satisfies the above criteria, though not exclusively.

9.1 Steps in analysis

1. Estimate the RER using replicate data. Screen replicates and flag those with anomalous errors.

2. When fitting the calibration curve use weighted least squares regression wherever possible.

3. Assess the fit of the model to the calibration data by analysis of variance (ANOVA).

4. Calculate the variance ratio of deviation from the model/replicate variance.

5. A minimum of eight dose levels is recommended for the calibration curve.

Assess between batch precision.

The guidelines have not been revised since they were published and it is generally accepted that six dose levels are adequate to form the calibration curve.

10 Diagnostic performance

10.1 Clinical sensitivity and specificity

The clinical sensitivity measures the detection of patients with the disease, it is the proportion of true positive the are correctly identified. This is also known as the detection rate.

Sensitivity (positivity in disease) = {(True positives)/(True positives = False negatives)} × 100.

The clinical specificity measures the detection of patients who do not have the disease, it is the proportion of true negatives that are correctly identified.

Specificity (negativity in health) = {(True positives)/(True negatives + False positives)} × 100.

6. Calculate the apparent concentration of analyte in the calibrators when treated as unknowns.
7. Combine the RER with the slope of the fitted calibration curve to estimate the error in concentration of unknowns.
8. Determine statistically the estimate of the minimum detectable concentration.
9. Report the unknowns with an estimate of their precision, this may be expressed as %CV from the precision profile or as 95% confidence limits. Flag those samples with errors greater than a fixed limit.
10. Calculate values for diluted samples within the assay.
11. Assess the assay for drift or instability by including the same samples in different positions in the assay.

9.2 Quality control

Use at least three quality control samples each with different analyte concentrations.

Monitor the performance of the quality controls on control charts.

Positive predictive value, this is the likelihood that a patient with a positive result actually has the disease, it is the proportion of patients with a positive test result who are correctly identified.

Predictive value of a positive result = {(True positives)/(True positives + False positives)} × 100.

Negative predictive value, this is the likelihood that a patient with a negative result does not have the disease, it is the proportion of patients with negative test results who are correctly identified.

Predictive value of a negative result = {(True negatives)/(True negatives = False negatives)} × 100.

10.2 Likelihood ratios

Positive likelihood ratio = sensitivity/(1 − specificity); negative likelihood ratio = specificity/(1 − sensitivity).

Data Processing

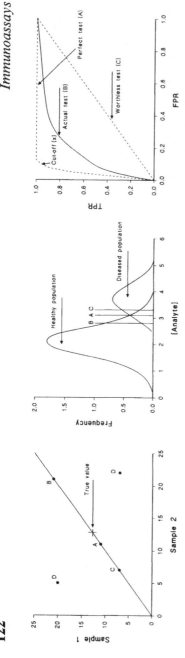

Figure 10. Youden plot for external QCs. The position of the points on the plot will define the performance characteristic of the assay in terms of bias and precision.

Figure 11. Selection of cut-off for a diagnostic test.

Figure 12. Receiver operator characteristics (ROC) curves. FPR, false positive rate; TPR, true positive rate.

10.3 Receiver operator characteristics (ROC) curves

To interpret a diagnostic test correctly, a cut-off point must be selected. The separates negatives from positives must be selected. The position of this cut-off will determine the level of incorrect nondiseased subjects at any cut-off point. Curve B represents an actual test with performance intermediate between the two extremes. ROC analysis is now an accepted and frequently reported method of determining the classification as healthy or diseased. If the cut-off is placed at A, there is a degree of overlap between diseased and nondiseased subjects. If the cut-off is moved to C fewer nondiseased subjects are misclassified, but more of the diseased population are incorrectly identified as nondiseased. If the cut-off is moved to B the situation is reversed (see *Figure 11*).

As previously defined, the true positive ratio + false negative ratio = 1; also the true negative ratio + false positive ratio = 1. Receiver operating characteristics (ROC) curves describe the way in which the two test properties (true positive ratio and false positive ratio) vary as the cut-off of a diagnostic test is varied. See *Figure 12*: in a near perfect test (curve A) most diseased and nondiseased subjects are identified correctly with the cut-off plotted at *x*. In a useless test (curve C) there is no separation of diseased and

performance of a diagnostic test and can be applied to all forms of diagnostic technologies.

10.4 Half-life calculation of tumor markers

Regular monitoring of circulating levels of tumor markers such as alphafetoprotein (AFP) can facilitate the calculation of the half-life of the marker in plasma after surgery.

Application of the equation

$$t_{\frac{1}{2}} = \frac{-0.3t_\Delta}{\log_{10}\frac{[AFP]T}{[AFP]T_0}}$$

where $t_{\frac{1}{2}}$ is the half-life; t_Δ is the difference in the days between sample on day T and earlier sample on day T_0; $[AFP]T$ concentration of marker on day T; $[AFP]T_0$ concentration of marker on day T_0.

Chapter 12 MANUFACTURERS AND SUPPLIERS

Nunc A/S, Kamstruprej 90, Postbox 280, Kamstrup, DK 4000, Roskilde, Denmark. Tel 46 35 90 65. Fax 46 35 01 05.

Microtiter plates (MTP)

Abbott Diagnostics Division, 100 Abbott Park Road, Abbott Park, North Chicago, IL 60064-3537, USA. Tel (708) 937 6100. Fax (708) 323 9100.
Abbott House, Norden Road, Maidenhead, Berks SL6 4XE, UK. Tel (01628) 784041. Fax (01628) 644305.

Automated immunoassay analyzer, e.g. IMX and Axsym

Alpha Laboratories, 40 Parham Drive, Eastleigh, Hants SO50 4NU, UK. Tel (01703) 610911. Fax (01703) 643701.

MTP readers

Anthos Labtec Instruments, Jakob-Haringer-Straße 8, Postfach 8, A-5022 Salzburg, Austria. Tel (0662) 454910. Fax (0662) 454914.

MTP equipment

Amersham International plc, Amersham Place, Little Chalfont, Bucks HP7 9NA, UK. Tel (01494) 544000. Fax (01494) 542266.
Amersham Corporation, 2636 South Clearbrook Drive, Arlington Heights, Il 60005, USA. Tel (708) 593 6300.

Radio labeled reagents and radioisotopes

Baxter Healthcare Ltd, Wallingford Road, Compton, Newbury, Berks RG16 7QW, UK. Tel (01635) 206000.

Automated analyzer, e.g. Stratus

Bayer Diagnostics, Bayer Plc, Evans House, Hamilton Close, Houndmills, Basingstoke, Hants RG21 6YE, Tel (01256) 29181. Fax (01256) 52916.

Automated analyzer, e.g. Technicon Immuno

Beckman Instruments (UK) Ltd, Oakley Court, Kingsmead Business Park, London Road, High Wycombe, Bucks HP11 1JU, UK. Tel (01494) 442233.

Automated analyzer

Becton Dickinson Corporation, Becton Drive, Franklin Lakes, NJ 07417-1880, USA. Tel (201) 847 6800. Fax (201) 847 6475. Between Towns Road, Cowley, Oxford OX4 3LY, UK. Tel (01865) 748844. Fax (01865) 717313.

Automated sample/reagent processor, e.g. Biomek 2000

Behring Diagnostics UK Ltd, Walton Manor, Walton, Milton Keynes, Bucks MK7 7AJ, UK. Tel (01908) 680567. Fax (01908) 680570.

Automated analyzer, e.g. Opus Magnum

151 University Avenue, Westwood, MA 02090, USA. Tel (617) 320 3000. Fax (617) 320 3085.

BioChem ImmunoSystems (UK) Ltd, 20 Woking Business Park, Albert Drive, Woking, Surrey GU21 5JY, UK. Tel (01483) 755330. Fax (01483) 755889.

Monoclonal antibodies, automated analyzer, e.g. SRI Immunoreagents

Biogenesis Ltd, 7 New Fields, Stinsford Road, Poole, Dorset BH17 0NF, UK. Tel (01202) 660006. Fax (01202) 660020.

bioMérieux sa, 69280 Marcy-l'Etoile, France. Tel 78 87 20 00. Fax 78 87 20 90. Grafton House, Grafton Way, Basingstoke, Hants, RG22 6HY, UK. Tel (01256) 461881. Fax (01256) 816863.

Automated analyzer, e.g. Vidas

Bio-Rad Laboratories Ltd, Bio-Rad House, Maylands Avenue, Hemel Hempstead, Herts HP2 7TD, UK. Tel (0800) 181134. Fax (01442) 259118. Alfred Nobel Drive, Hercules, CA 94547. USA. Tel (510) 741 1000. Fax (510) 741 1060.

Automated analyzer, e.g. Radias Quality Control material

Boehringer Mannheim Corporation, 9115 Hague Road, PO Box 50446, Indianapolis, IN 46250-0446, USA. Tel (317) 845 2000. Boehringer Mannheim UK (Diagnostics & Biochemicals) Ltd, Bell Lane, Lewes, East Sussex BN7 1LG, UK. Tel (01273) 480444.

Automated analyzer, e.g. ES 300

Manufacturers and Suppliers

Byk-Sangtec Diagnostica GmbH & Co. KG, von Hevesy-Straße 3, 63128, Dietzenbach, Germany. Tel (6074) 4010. Fax (6074) 401209.

Automated analyzer, e.g. LiaMat and RiaMat

Canberra Packard Instrument Company, 800 Research Parkway, Meriden, CT 06450, USA. Tel (203) 238 2351. Fax (203) 235 1347.

Automated sample/reagent processor and scintillation counters

Chemicon International Ltd, 2 Bonnersfield Lane, Harrow, Middx, HA1 2JR, UK. Tel (0181) 863 0415. Fax (0181) 863 0416. 28835 Single Oak Drive, Temecula, CA 92590, USA. Tel (909) 676 8080. Fax (909) 676 9209.

Monoclonals

Ciba Corning Diagnostics Ltd, Colchester Road, Halstead, Essex CO9 2DX, UK. Tel (01787) 472461. Fax (01787) 475088. Worldwide Corporate Headquarters, 63 North Street, Medfield, MA 02052, USA. Tel (508) 359 3807. Fax (508) 359 3879.

Automated analyzer, e.g. ACS 180

CIS (UK) Ltd, Dowding House, Wellington Road, High Wycombe, Bucks HP12 3PR, UK. Tel (01494) 535922. Fax (01494) 521785. CIS US, Inc., 10 De Angelo Drive, Bedford, MA, 01730, USA. Tel (617) 275 7120. Fax (617) 275 2634.

Immunoreagents, radiolabeled reagents

Corning Costar Corporation, One Alewife Center, Cambridge, MA 02140, USA. Tel (617) 868 6200. Fax (617) 868 2076. Costar UK Ltd, 10 The Valley Centre, Gordon Road, High Wycombe, Bucks HP13 6EQ, UK. Tel (01494) 471207. Fax (01494) 464891.

Microtiter plates

Diagnostics Products Corporation, 5700 West 96th Street, Los Angeles, CA 90045-5597, USA. Tel (213) 776 0180/(800) 372 1782. Fax (213) 776 0204. DPL Division, EURO/DPC Ltd, Glyn Rhonwy, Llanberis, Caernarfon, Gwynedd

Automated analyzer, e.g. Immulite

LL55 4EL, UK. Tel (01286) 871872. Fax (01286) 871794.
5700 West 96th Street, Los Angeles, CA, 90045, USA. Tel (213) 773 0180.
DuPont NEN (UK) Ltd, Wedgewood Way, Stevenage, Hert SG1 4QN, UK. Tel (01438) 73 40 27. Fax (01438) 73 4379.
949 Albany Street, Boston, MA 02118, USA. Tel (617) 482 9595. Fax (617) 542 8463.

Radiolabeled immunoreagents/automated analyzer, e.g. aCa plus

Dynatech Laboratories, Duax Road, Billingshurst, West Sussex RH14 9SJ, UK. Tel (01403) 783381. Fax (01403) 784397.
14340 Sullyfield Circle, Chantilly, VA 22021, USA. Tel (703) 631 7800. Fax (703) 803 1441.

Automated MTP processors, e.g. DIAS

EG&G Ltd Milton Keynes comprising Wallac (UK) and Berthold (UK) operations, 20 Vincent Avenue, Crownhill Business Centre, Crownhill, Milton Keynes MK8 0AB, UK. Tel (01908) 265744. Fax (01908) 265956/265989.

Automated analyzer, e.g. DELFIA/data processing software/counters

Eurogenetics UK Ltd, Unit 5, Kingsway Business Park, Oldfield Road, Hampton TW12 2HD, UK. Tel (0181) 296 8800. Fax (0181) 296 9039.
TOSOH Corporation, TOSOH KYOBASHI Building, 2–4, 3-Chome, Kyobashi, Chuo-ku, Tokyo, Japan. Tel (3) 3275 1061. Fax (3) 3275 1214.

Automated analyzer, e.g. Tosoh 1200

Fitzgerald Industries International Inc, 34 Junction Square Drive, Concord, MA 01742-3049, USA. Tel (508) 371 6446. Fax (508) 371 2266.

Antisera and monoclonals

Genzyme Corporation, One Kendall Square, Cambridge, MA 02139-1562 USA. Tel (617) 252 7500. Fax (617) 252 7759.
Genzyme Diagnostics, 50 Gibson Drive, Kings Hill, West Malling, Kent ME19 6HG, UK. Tel (01732) 220022. Fax (01732) 220024/5.

Immunoreagents

Guildhay Ltd, 6 Riverside Business Centre, Walnut Tree Close, Guildford, Surrey GU1 4UG, UK. Tel (01483) 573727. Fax (01483) 574828.

Antisera

Hamilton (GB) Ltd, Unit Z, Lyne Riggs Estate, Lancaster Road, Carnforth, Lancs LA5 9EA, UK. Tel (01524) 720650. Fax (01524) 720651.
PO Box 10 030, Reno, NV 89520, USA. Tel (702) 858 3000. Fax (702) 856 7259.

Automated processors, e.g. Fame PTTP

Harlan Bioproducts for Science, Inc., PO Box 29176, Indianapolis, IN 46229–0176, USA. Tel (317) 894 7536. Fax (317) 894 1840.
Harlan Sera-Lab Ltd, Crawley Down, Sussex RH10 4FF, UK. Tel (01342) 716366. Fax (01342) 717351.

Immunoreagents

ICN Biomedicals Inc, 3300 Hyland Avenue, Costa Mesa CA 92626, USA.
Tel (800) 854 0530. Fax (800) 854 0530.
Unit 18, Thame Park Business Centre, Winman Road, Thame, Oxon OX9 3XA, UK.
Tel (0800) 282474/(01844) 213366. Fax (0800) 614735/(01844) 213399.

Radiolabeled agents

Immunodiagnostic Systems Ltd, Boldon Business Park, Boldon, Tyne & Wear NE35 9PD, UK. Tel (0191) 519 0660. Fax (0191) 519 0760.

Solid phase second antibodies (SacCel)

Incstar Ltd, Charles House, Toutley Road, Wokingham, Berks RG41 1QN, UK.
Tel (01734) 772693. Fax (01734) 792061.

Immunoreagents

Johnson & Johnson Clinical Diagnostics, 100 Indigo Creek Drive, Rochester, NY 14650, USA. Tel (716) 453 3390.
Mandeville House, 62 The Broadway, Amersham, Bucks HP7 0HJ, UK.
Tel (01494) 431717. Fax (01494) 431165.

Automated analyzer, e.g. Amerlite

The Kemble Instrument Company Ltd, Marchants Way, Burgess Hill, West Sussex RH15 8QY, UK. Tel (0144) 871187. Fax (0144) 871088.

Automated sample/reagent processor, e.g. Guardian

Labsystems Oy, PO Box 8, 3F-00881, Helsinki, Finland. Tel 0 75821. Fax 0 755 524.

MTP readers

Lab Tech International, Woodside, Easons Green, Uckfield, West Sussex TN22 5RE, UK. Tel (01825) 840024. Fax (01825) 841112.

MTP readers

Librapharm Ltd, Gemini House, 162 Craven Road, Newbury, Berks RG14 5NR, UK. Tel (01635) 522651. Fax (01635) 522651.

Directory for sources of diagnostic kits

Life Science International, Unit 5, The Ringway Centre, Edison Road, Basingstoke, Hants RG21 2YH, UK. Tel (01256) 817 282. Fax (01256) 817292.

MTP automated equipment

Linscott's Directory, 40 Glen Drive, Mill Valley, CA 94941, USA. Tel (415) 383 2666.

Directory of international sources of antibodies

Molecular Probes Inc., PO Box 22010, Eugene, OR 97402-0414, USA. Tel (541) 465 8338. Fax (541) 344 6504.

Fluorescent molecular probes

Molecular Probes Europe BV, Poort Gebouw, Rijnsburgerweg 10, 2333 AA Leiden, The Netherlands. Tel (71) 5 233378. Fax (71) 5 233419.

Organon Teknika nv, Veedijk 58, 2300 Tournhout, Belgium. Tel (14) 40 40 40. Fax (14) 42 16 00.

Automated analyzer, e.g. Auraflex

Packard Instrument Company, 800 Research Parkway, Meriden, CT 06450, USA. Tel (800) 323 1891/(203) 238 2351. Fax (203) 639 2172.

Automated equipment – processors and counters (radio)

The Perkin Elmer Corporation, 761 Main Avenue, Norwalk, CT 06859-0012, USA. Tel (203) 762 1000/(800) 762 8288. Fax (203) 761 5057.

Fluorometers

Pharmacia Biotechnology, 23 Grosvenor Road, St Albans, Herts AL1 3AW, UK. Tel (01727) 814000. Fax (01727) 814020.
800 Centennial Avenue, PO Box 1327, Piscataway, NJ 08855-1327, USA. Tel 201 457 8000. Fax 201 457 0557.

Immunosupports and chromatographic supports

Manufacturers and Suppliers

Pierce & Warriner (UK) Ltd, 44 Upper Northgate Street, Chester CH1 4EF, UK.
Tel (01244) 382525. Fax (01244) 373212.

Antisera

Pierce, Perstorp Biotec, 3747 N Meridian Road, PO Box 117, Rockford, Il 61105, USA.
Tel (800) 874 3723/(815) 968 0747. Fax (815) 968 7316.

Antisera

Polyclonal Antibodies Ltd, Blaenwaun Farm, Ffostrasol, nr. Llandysul, Dyfed SA44 5JT,
UK. Tel (01239) 851378. Fax (01239) 858800.

Polyclonal antisera, contract
antisera

Quatro Biosystems Ltd, Probus House, Broadoak Business Centre, Ashburton Road
West, Manchester M17 1RW, UK. Tel (0161) 848 0300. Fax (0161) 848 0157.

Automated sample/reagent
processor, e.g. SP 240

Robert Maciel Associates Inc, 870 Massachusetts Avenue, PO Box 212, Arlington,
MA 02174-0002, USA. Tel (617) 646 3627. Fax (617) 648 7607.

Software – data reduction

Roche Diagnostics, CH-4002 Basel, Switzerland, Tel (61) 687 2400.
Fax (61) 687 2848.
PO Box 8, Welwyn Garden City, Hertfordshire AL7 3AY, UK. Tel (01707) 366735.
Fax (01707) 373556.

Automated analyzer, e.g. Cobas Core

Rosys Ag, Feldbachstrasse, CH-8634, Hombrechtikon, Switzerland. Tel (55) 254 2111.
Fax (55) 254 2100.

Automated processors, e.g. Plato
3300

Scantibodies Laboratory Inc., 9336 Abraham Way, Santee, CA 92071, USA.
Tel (619) 258 9300. Fax (619) 258 9366.

Sera, antisera

SCIPAC Ltd, Broad Oak Road, Sittingbourne, Kent ME9 8AQ, UK.
Tel (01795) 423077. Fax (01795) 426942.

Immunoreagents and solid phase

Scottish Antibody Production Unit, Law Hospital, Carluke, Lanarks, ML8 5ES, UK.
Tel (01698) 351161. Fax (01698) 359376.

Antisera, contact antisera and
monoclonals

Scripps Laboratories Inc., 6838 Flanders Drive, San Diego, CA 92121-2904, USA.
Tel (619) 546 5800. Fax (619) 546 5812.

Antisera and monoclonals

Serotec, 22 Bankside, Station Field Industrial Estate, Kidlington, Oxford OX5 1JE, UK.
Tel (01865) 379941. Fax (01865) 373899.

Immunoreagents

Sigma Diagnostics, Fancy Road, Poole, Dorset BH17 4QH, UK. Tel (0800) 373731.
Fax (01202) 715460.
PO Box 14508, St Louis, MI 63178, USA. Tel (314) 771 5765. Fax (314) 771 5757.

Antisera, immunoreagents

SLT Labinstruments GmbH, Untersbergstrasse 1A, E-5082 Grödig, Salzburg, Austria.
Tel (6246) 8933. Fax (6246) 72770.

Automated processors

TCS Biologicals Ltd, Botolph Claydon, Buckingham MK18 2LR, UK.
Tel (01296) 714071. Fax (01296) 714806.

Immunoreagents, contract antisera

Tecan UK Ltd, 18 The High Street, Goring on Thames, Reading, Berks UK.
Tel (01491) 875087. Fax (01491) 875 432.

Automated sample/reagent processors, e.g. Genesis

Manufacturers and Suppliers

REFERENCES

Chapter 1

1. Uhlenhuth, T. (1903) *Dtsch. Med. Wschr.* **29**, 39.
2. Bechhold, H. (1905) *Z. Phys. Chem.* **52**, 185.
3. Landsteiner, K. (1943) *The Specificity of Serological Reactions*. Harvard University Press, Cambridge, MA.
4. Heidelberger, M. (1929) *J. Exp. Med.* **50**, 809
5. Coons, A.H. *et al.* (1941) *Proc. Soc. Exp. Biol. Med.* **47**, 200.
6. Oudin, J. (1946) *C.R. Acad. Sci.* **222**, 115.
7. Ouchterlony, Ö. (1948) *Acta. Pathol. Microbiol. Scand.* **25**, 186.
8. Arquila, E.R. and Statvitsky, A.B. (1956) *J. Clin. Invest.* **35**, 458.
9. Ekins, R.P. (1960) *Clin. Chim. Acta.* **5**, 453.
10. Yalow, R.S. and Berson, S.A. (1960) *J. Clin. Invest.* **39**, 1157.
11. Wide, L. *et al.* (1967) *Lancet* **2**, 1105.
12. Miles, L.E.M. and Hales, C.N. (1968) *Nature* **219**, 186.
13. Haberman, E. (1970) *Z. Klin. Chem. Klin. Biochem.* **8**, 51.
14. Wide, L. (1971) in *Radioimmunoassay Methods* (K.E. Kirkham and W.M. Hunter, eds), p. 405. Churchill Livingstone, Edinburgh.

2. Ekins R.P. (1991) in *Principles and Practice of Immunoassays* (C.P. Price and D.J. Newman, eds), p. 96. Macmillan, London and Stockton Press, New York.
3. Jackson T.M. and Ekins R.P. (1986) *J. Immunol. Meth.* **87**, 13.
4. Ekins, R.P. (1983) in *Immunoassays for Clinical Chemistry*, 2nd Edn (W.M. Hunter and J.E.T. Corrie, eds), p. 76. Churchill Livingstone, Edinburgh.

Chapter 4

1. Monji, N. and Castro, A. (1979) *Res. Commun. Chem. Pathol. Pharmacol.* **26**, 187.
2. Ullman, E.F. *et al.* (1975) *Clin. Chem.* **21**, 1011.
3. Dandliker, W.B. and Feigen, G. (1961) *Biochem. Biophys. Res. Commun.* **5**, 299.
4. Shaw, E.J. *et al.* (1977) *J. Clin. Pathol.* **30**, 526.
5. Smith, D.S. (1977) *FEBS Lett.* **77**, 25.

15. Addison, G.M. and Hales, C.N. (1971) *Horm. Metab. Res.* **3**, 59.
16. Kohler, G. and Milstein, C. (1975) *Nature* **256**, 495.

Chapter 2

1. Edwards R. (1990) *Radioimmunoassay*, p. 71. IRL Press, Oxford.
2. Siddle, K. (1990) in *Peptide Hormone Secretion* (J.C. Hutton and K. Siddle, eds.). p. 97. IRL Press, Oxford University Press, Oxford.
3. Kohler G. and Milstein C. (1975) *Nature* **256**, 495.
4. Abraham, G.E. (1968) *J. Clin. Endocr. Metab.* **29**, 866.
5. Edwards R. and Rees L.H. (1994) in *Diagnostic tests in Endocrinology and Diabetes* (P.-M.G. Boulox and L.H. Rees, eds.), p.1. Chapman & Hall Medical, London.
6. Hurn, B.A.L. and Chantler, S.M. (1980) *Meth. Enzymol.* **70**, 104.
7. Edwards, R. et al. (1992) in *Developments in Radioimmunoassay and Related Procedures*, p. 205. Proceedings Symposium, Vienna 1991. International Atomic Energy Agency, Vienna.
8. Mage M.G. (1980) *Meth. Enzymol.* **70**, 142.

Chapter 3

1. Ekins R.P. (1976) in *General Principles of Hormone Assay* (J.H. Loraine and E.T. Bell, eds.), p. 1. Churchill Livingstone, Edinburgh.

6. Nargessi, R.D. and Landon, J. (1981) *Meth. Enzymol.* **74**, 60.
7. Ullman, E.F. and Khanna, P.L. (1981) *Meth. Enzymol.* **74**, 28.
8. Bosworth, N. and Towers, P. (1989) *Nature* **341**, 167.
9. Axelson, N.H. (1983) *Handbook of Immunoprecipitation in Gel Techniques.* Blackwell Scientific Publications, Oxford.
10. Coombs, R.A.A. *et al.* (1987) *J. Immunol. Meth.* **101**, 1.
11. Price, C.P. and Newman, D.J. (eds) (1991) *Principles and Practice of Immunoassays*, p. 446. Macmillan, London and Stockton Press, New York.
12. Yalow, R.S. and Berson, S. (1960) *J. Clin. Invest.* **39**, 1157.
13. Ekins, R.P. (1960) *Clin. Chem. Acta.* **5**, 453.
14. Giese, J. *et al.* (1970) *Scand. J. Clin. Lab. Invest.* **26**, 355.
15. Odell, W.D. (1980) *Meth. Enzymol.* **70**, 274.
16. Johansson, E.D.B. (1970) *Acta Endocrinol. Suppl.* **147**, 188.
17. Trafford, D.J.H. and Makin, H. L. J. (1980) *Meth. Enzymol.* **70**, 291.
18. Chard, T. (1980) *Meth. Enzymol.* **70**, 280.
19. Morgan, C.R. and Lazarow, A. (1962) *Proc. Soc. Exp. Biol. Med.* **110**, 29.
20. Midgley, J.R. and Hepburn, M.R. (1980) *Meth. Enzymol.* **70**, 266.
21. Edwards, R. (1983) in *Immunoassays in Clinical Chemistry* (W. M. Hunter and J.E.T. Corrie, eds), p. 139. Churchill Livingstone, Edinburgh.
22. Catt, K.J. and Tregear, G.W. (1967) *Science*, **158**, 1570.

23. Bangs, L.B. (1984) *Uniform Latex Particles*. Seradyn Inc., PO Box 1210, IN, USA.

24. Edwards, R. (1990) *Radioimmunoassay*, p. 71. IRL Press, Oxford.

25. Hendry, R.M. and Herriman, J.E. (1980) *J. Immunol. Meth.* **35**, 285.

26. Line, W.F. and Becker, M.J. (1975) in *Immobilised Enzymes, Antigens, Antibodies and Peptides* (H.H. Weetall, ed.), p. 285. Marcel Dekker, New York.

27. Forrest, G.C. and Rattle, S.J. (1983) in *Immunoassays in Clinical Chemistry* (W.M. Hunter and J.E.T. Corrie, eds), p. 147. Churchill Livingstone, Edinburgh.

28. Weetall, H.H. (1976) *Meth. Enzymol.* **44**, 134.

29. Nustad, K. *et al.* (1984) *Eur. Surg. Res.* **16**, Suppl 2, 80.

30. Donini, S. *et al.* (1968) in *Gonadotrophins* (Rosenberg, ed.). Los Altes, CA, USA.

31. Goodfriend, T.L. *et al.* (1969) *Immunochemistry* **6**, 481.

32. Lim, F. and Buehler, R.J. (1981) *Meth. Enzymol.* **73**, 254.

33. Diamandis, E.P. and Christopoulos, T.K. (1991) *Clin. Chem.* **37**, 625.

34. Wide, L. (1981) *Meth. Enzymol.* **73**, 203.

35. Nilsson, K. and Mosbach, K. (1980) *Eur. J. Biochem.* **112**, 397.

36. Nilsson, K. and Mosbach, K. (1981) *Biochem. Biophys. Res.* **102**, 449.

37. Chapman, R.S. *et al.* (1983) in *Immunoassays in Clinical Chemistry*

4. Engvall, E. and Perlmann, P. (1971) *Immunochemistry* **8**, 871.

5. van Weeman, B.K. and Schuurs, A.H.W.M. (1971) *FEBS Lett.* **15**, 232.

6. Rubenstein, K.E. *et al.* (1972) *Biochem. Biophys. Res. Commun.* **47**, 846.

7. Sevier, E.D. *et al.* (1981) *Clin. Chem.* **27**, 1797.

8. Enzyme Commission (1979) *Enzyme Nomenclature*. Academic Press, NY.

9. Welinder, K.G. (1979) *Eur. J. Biochem.* **96**, 483.

10. Neumann, H. and Lustig, A. (1980) *Eur. J. Biochem.* **109**, 475.

11. McComb, R.B. and Bowers, G.N. (eds), (1979) in *Alkaline Phosphatase*, p. 175. Plenum Press, New York.

12. Rothman, F. and Byrne, R. (1963) *J. Mol. Biol.* **6**, 330.

13. Fowler, A.V. and Zabin, I. (1977) *Proc. Natl Acad. Sci. USA* **74**, 1507.

14. Nakamura, S. *et al.* (1976) in *Flavin and Flavoproteins* (T.P. Singer, ed.) p. 691. Elsevier/North Holland, Amsterdam.

15. Bergmeyer, H.-U. (ed.) (1974) *Methods of Enzymatic Analysis*, Vol. 1–4. Academic Press, New York.

16. Canfield, R.E. *et al.* (1974) in *Lysozyme* (E.F. Osserman, R.E. Canfield, and S. Beychock, eds) p. 63. Academic Press, New York.

17. Banaszak, L.J. and Bradshaw, R.A. (1975) in *The Enzymes* (P.D. Boyer, ed.), Vol 11, p. 369. Academic Press, New York.

18. Milhausen, M. and Levy, H.R. (1975) *Biochemistry* **5**, 453.

(W.M. Hunter and J.E.T. Corrie, eds), p. 178. Churchill Livingstone, Edinburgh.

Chapter 5

1. Morgan, C.R. (1966) *Proc. Soc. Exp. Biol. Med.* **123**, 230.
2. Edwards R. (1990) *Radioimmunoassay*, p. 71. IRL Press, Oxford.
3. Bolton, A.E. and Hunter, W.M. (1973) *Biochem. J.* **133**, 529.
4. Edwards, R. *et al.* (1992) in *Proceedings Symposium, Vienna 1991*, p. 205. International Atomic Energy Agency, Vienna.
5. Thorell, J.I. *et al.* (1982) in *Radioimmunoassay and Related Procedures in Medicine*, p.147. International Atomic Energy Agency, Vienna.
6. Linde, S. *et al.* (1983) *Adv. Enzymol.* **92**, 309.
7. Hales, C.N. and Woodhead, J.S. (1980) *Adv. Enzymol.* **70**, 334.

Chapter 6

1. Avrameas, S. and Uriel, J. (1966) *Compt. Rend. Acad. Sci. Paris* **265**, 1149.
2. Nakane, N.K. and Pierce, G.B. (1966) *J. Histochem. Cytochem.* **14**, 929.
3. Nakane, N.K. and Pierce, G.B. (1967) *J. Cell. Biol.* **33**, 307.
19. Tiggerman, R. *et al.* (1981) *J. Histochem. Cytochem.* **29**, 1387.
20. Saunders, B.C. *et al.* (1964) in *Peroxidase*, p. 271. Butterworths, London.
21. Marklund, S. (1973) *Arch. Biochem. Biophys.* **154**, 614.
22. McCracken, S. and Meighen, E.A. (1981) *J. Biol. Chem.* **256**, 3945.
23. Caswell, M. and Caplow, M. (1980) *Biochemistry* **19**, 2907.
24. Bentley, R. (1963) in *The Enzymes* (P.D. Boyer *et al.*, eds), Vol. 7, p. 567. Academic Press, New York.
25. Peterson, J. *et al.* (1948) *J. Biol. Chem.* **176**, 1.
26. Olive, C. and Levy, H.R. (1971) *J. Biol. Chem.* **245**, 2043.
27. Rowley, G.L. *et al.* (1975) *J. Biol. Chem.* **250**, 3759.
28. Bergmeyer, H.-U. (ed.) (1963) in *Methods of Enzymatic Analysis*, 2nd Edn, p. 783. Academic Press, New York.
29. Moessner, E. *et al.* (1980) *Hoppe-Seyler's Z. Physiol. Chem.* **361**, 543.
30. Willstatter, R and Stoll, A. (1917) *Liebigs Ann. Chem.* **416**, 21.
31. Makinen, K.K. and Tenovuo, J. (1982) *Anal. Biochem.* **126**, 100.
32. Hildebrandt, A.G. and Roots, I. (1975) *Arch. Biochem. Biophys.* **171**, 385.
33. Mahler *et al* (1948) *J. Biol. Chem.* **179**, 961.
34. Lohr, G.W. and Waller, H.D. (1974) in *Methods of Enzymatic Analysis* (H.-U. Bergmeyer, ed.), p. 636. Academic Press, New York.
35. Sumner, J.B. (1955) *Meth. Enzymol.* **2**, 378.

36. Shugar, D. (1952) *Biochim. Biophys. Acta* **8**, 302.
37. Means, G.E. and Feeney, R.E. (1990) *Bioconjugate Chem.* **1**, 2
38. Kennedy, J.H. *et al.* (1976) *Clin. Chim. Acta* **70**, 1.
39. Lomants, A.J. and Fairbanks, G. (1976) *Arch. Biochem. Biophys.* **167**, 311.
40. Duncan, R.J.S. *et al.* (1983) *Anal. Biochem.* **132**, 68.
41. Jue, R. *et al.* (1978) *Biochemistry* **17**, 5399.
42. Nakane, P.K. and Kawaoi, A. (1974) *J. Histochem. Cytochem.* **22**, 1084.
43. Tijssen, P. and Kurstak. E. (1984) *Anal. Biochem.* **136**, 451.
44. Yoshitake, S. (1983) *J. Biochem.* **92**, 1413.
45. Avrameas, S. and Ternynck, T. (1971) *Immunochemistry* **8**, 1175.
46. Halpern, E.P. *et al* (1972) *Clin. Chem.* **18**, 593.
47. Blake, M.S. *et al.* (1984) *Anal. Biochem.* **136**, 175.
48. Bos, E.S. *et al.* (1981) *J. Immunoassay* **2**, 187.
49. Boviard, J.H. *et al.* (1982) *J. Clin. Chem.* **28**, 2423.
50. Avrameas, S. and Guilbert, B. (1976) *Biochimie* **54**, 837.
51. Gallati, H (1979) *J. Clin. Chem. Clin. Biochem.* **17**, 1.
52. Ellens, D.J. and Gielkins, A.L.J. (1980) *J. Immunol. Meth.* **37**, 325.
53. Barile, F. and Trombetta, L.D. (1982) *J. Histochem.* **5**, 12.
54. Kaplow, L.S. *et al.* (1974) *Am J. Clin. Path.* **63**, 451.
55. Tanimori, H. et al. (1983) *J. Immunol. Meth.* **62**, 123.
56. Self, C.H. (1985) *J. Immunol. Meth.* **76**, 389.

20. Siepak, J. (1989) *Analyst.* **114**, 529.
21. Beverloo, H. B. *et al.* (1992) *Anal. Biochem.* **203**, 326.
22. Blincko, S. (1989) *Novel luminescent compounds for immunoassay.* PhD thesis, The City University, London.
23. Haughland, R.P. (1983) in *Excited States of Biopolymers* (R.F. Steiner, ed.), p. 29. Plenum Press, New York.
24. Dandliker, W.B. and Portmann, A.J. (1971) in *Excited States of Proteins and Nucleic Acids* (R.F. Steiner and I. Weinryb, eds), Plenum Press, New York.
25. Huang, Z. (1991) *Biochemistry* **30**, 8530.
26. Goding, J.W. (1976) *J. Immunol. Meth.* **13**, 215.
27. Viinikka, L. *et al.* (1981) *Clin. Chim. Acta.* **114**, 1.
28. Eremin, S.A. *et al.* (1988) *Therap. Drug Monit.* **10**, 327.
29. Carlsson, J. *et al.* (1978) *Biochem. J.* **173**, 723.
30. Parker, C.A. (1968) *The Photoluminescence of Solutions.* Elsevier, Amsterdam.
31. Williams, W.P. (1983) in *Biochemical Research Techniques* (J.M. Wrigglesworth, ed.). John Wiley & Sons, New York.

Chapter 8

1. Campbell, A.K. (1988) *Chemiluminescence Principles and Applications in Biology and Medicine.* Ellis Horwood, Chichester.

Chapter 7

1. Soini, E. and Hemmilla, I. (1979) *Clin. Chem.* **25**, 353.
2. Hemmila, I. (1985) *Clin. Chem.* **31**, 359.
3. Hemmila, I., Stahlberg, T. and Mottram, P. (1994) *Bioanalytical Applications of Labelling Technologies*. Wallac. Finland.
4. Sidki, A.M. and Landon, J. (1985) in *Alternative Immunoassays* (W. P. Collins and J. Wiley, eds), p.185. John Wiley & Sons, New York.
5. Hemmila, I. *et al.* (1988) *Clin. Chem.* **34**, 2320.
6. Barnard, G. *et al.* (1989) *Clin. Chem.* **35**, 555.
7. Shaw, E.J. *et al.* (1977) *J. Clin. Pathol.* **30**,526.
8. Smith, D.S. (1977) *FEBS Lett.* **77**, 25.
9. Kronick, M. N. (1983) *Clin. Chem.* **29**,1582.
10. Ullman, E.F. *et al.* (1976) *J. Biol. Chem.* **251**, 4172.
11. Hassan, M. *et al.* (1982) *J. Immunoassay* **3**,1.
12. Zuk, R.F. *et al.* (1979) *Clin. Chem.* **25**, 1554.
13. Nargessi, R.D. *et al.* (1979) *J. Immunol. Meths.* **26**, 307.
14. Chen, R.F. (1969) *Arch. Biochem. Biophys.* **133**, 263.
15. *Handbook of Fluorescent Probes and Research Chemicals 1992–1994* (R.P. Haughland, ed.). Molecular Probes Inc. (see Chapter 12).
16. Kronick, M.N. (1986) *J. Immunol. Meth.* **92**, 1.
17. Chen, R.F. and Scott, C.H. (1985) *Anal. Lett.* **18**, 393.
18. McKinney, R.M. and Spillane,J.T. (1975) *Ann. N.Y. Acad. Sci.* **254**, 35.
19. Bailey, M.P. *et al.* (1985) *Analyst.* **110**, 603.

2. Price, C.P. and Newman, D.J. (eds) (1991) *Principles and Practice of Immunoassay*. Macmillan, London and Stockton Press, New York.
3. Kricka, L.J. (1991) *Clin. Chem.* **37**, 1472.
4. Kricka, L.J. and Thorpe, G.H.G. (1986) *Meth. Enzymol.* **133**, 404.
5. Barnard, G.J.R. *et al.* (1985) in *Alternative Immunoassays* (W.P. Collins, ed.), p. 123. John Wiley & Sons, New York.
6. Kohen, F. *et al.* (1985) in *Alternative Immunoassays* (W.P. Collins, ed.), p. 103. John Wiley & Sons, New York.
7. Carrico, R.J. *et al.* (1976) *Anal. Biochem.* **76**, 95.
8. Schroeder, H.R. *et al.* (1976) *Anal. Biochem.* **72**, 283.
9. Thorpe, G.H.G. and Kricka, L.J. (1987) in *Bioluminescence and Chemiluminescence – New Perspectives* (J. Schölmerich *et al.*, eds), p. 199. John Wiley & Sons, New York.
10. Kohen, F. *et al.* (1980) *Steroids* **36**, 29.
11. Campbell, A.K. *et al.* (1985) in *Alternative Immunoassays* (W.P. Collins, ed.), p. 153. John Wiley & Sons, New York.
12. Kricka, L.J. (1994) *Clin. Chem.* **40**, 347.
13. Shapiro, R. *et al.* (1984) *Clin. Chem.* **30**, 889.
14. Visenko, S.B. *et al.* (1989) *J. Biolumin. Chemilumin.* **4**, 164.
15. Miska, W. and Geiger, R. (1990) *J. Biolumin. Chemilumin.* **4**, 119.
16. Miska, W. and Geiger, R. (1987) *J. Clin. Chem. Clin. Biochem.* **25**, 23.
17. Bronstein, I. *et al.* (1990) *J. Biolumin. Chemilumin.* **4**, 99.
18. Bronstein, I. *et al.* (1989) *Clin. Chem.* **35**, 1441.

19. Bronstein, I. (1990) *U.S. Patent 4978614.*
20. Schaap, A.P. et al. (1989) *Clin. Chem.* **35**, 1863.
21. Motsenbacker, M. et al. (1993) *Anal. Chem.* **65**, 397.
22. Der-Ballen, G. P. et al. (1985) *European Patent Application 141581.*
23. Baldwin, T.O. et al. (1987) in *Bioluminescence and Chemiluminescence – New Perspectives* (J. Schölmerich et al., eds), p. 215. John Wiley & Sons, New York.
24. Lindbladh, C. et al. (1991) *J. Immunol. Meth.* **137**, 199.
25. Tsuji, A. et al. (1987) *Bioluminescence and Chemiluminescence – New Perspectives* (J. Schölmerich et al., eds), p. 233. John Wiley & Sons, New York.
26. Baret, A. et al. 90) *Anal. Biochem.* **187**, 20.
27. Baret, A. and Fert, V. (1990) *J. Biolumin. Chemilumin.* **4**, 149.
28. Tanaka, K. and Ishikaura, E. (1986) *Anal. Letts.* **19**, 433.
29. Hummelon, J.C. et al. (1986) *Meth. Enzymol.* **133**, 531.

22. Gribnau, T.C.J. et al. (1986) *J. Chromatography* **76**, 175.
23. Coombs R.R.A. (1981) in *Immunoassays for the 80's* (A. Voller, ed.), p. 17. MTP Press, Lancaster.
24. Coombs R.R.A. et al. (1987) *J. Immunol. Meth.* **101**, 1.
25. Binns, R.M. et al. (1982) *Immunology* **47**, 717.
26. Lemieux S. et al. (1974) *Immunochem.* **11**, 261.
27. Clark, M.R. (1986) *Meth. Enzymol.* **121**, 548.
28. Boyden, S.V. (1951) *J. Exp. Med.* **93**, 107.
29. Whitcher, J.T. and Blow, C. (1980) *Ann. Clin. Biochem.* **17**, 170.
30. Hechemy, K. et al. (1976) *J. Clin. Microbiol.* 4, 82.
31. Strutt, J.W. Rt Hon. (Lord Rayleigh) (1871) *Phil. Mag.* **41**, 447.
32. Debye, P. (1915) *Ann. Physik.* **46**, 809.
33. Mie, G. (1908) *Ann. Physik.* **25**, 377.
34. Maclin, E. et al. (1973) *Clin. Chem.* **19**, 832.
35. Price, C.P. and Spencer, K. (1981) *Clin. Chem.* **27**, 882.
36. Wood, P.J. et al. (1978) *Clin. Chim. Acta* **90**, 87.
37. Kallner, A. (1977) *Clin. Chim. Acta* **80**, 293.
38. Killingsworth L.M. and Savory, J. (1973) *Clin. Chem.* **19**, 403.
39. Whitcher, J.T. et al. (1982) *CRC Crit. Rev. Clin. Lab. Sci.* **18**, 213.
40. Wilkins, T.A. et al. (1988) in *Complimentary Immunoassays* (W.P. Collins, ed.), p. 227.
41. Masson, P.L. et al. (1981) *Methods Enzymol.* **74**, 106.
42. Bloomfield, V.A. (1985) in *Dynamic Light Scattering. Applications of Photon Correlation Spectroscopy*, p. 363. Plenum Press, New York.

Chapter 9

1. Heidelberger, M. and Kendall, F.W. (1935) *J. Exp. Med.* **62**, 467.
2. Hudson, L. and Hay, F.C. (1980) *Practical Immunology*, 2nd Edn. Blackwell Scientific Publications, Oxford.
3. Thorpe, R. and Johnstone A. (1982) *Immunochemistry in Practice.* Blackwell Scientific Publications, Oxford.
4. Mancini, G. et al. (1965) *Immunochemistry* **2**, 235.

5. Mancini, G. et al. (1970) Immunochemistry 7, 261.
6. Ouchterlony O. (1967) in Handbook of Experimental Immunology (D.M. Weir, ed.), p. 655. Blackwell Scientific Publications, Oxford.
7. Ouchterlony O. and Nilsson, L.-A. (1978) in Handbook of Experimental Immunology (D.M. Weir, ed.), 3rd Edn, p. 19. Blackwell Scientific Publications, Oxford.
8. Nilsson, L.-A. (1983) in Handbook of Immunoprecipitation-in-Gel Techniques (N.H. Axelsen, ed.), p. 71. Blackwell Scientific Publications, Oxford.
9. Clausen, J. (1969) in Laboratory Techniques in Biochemistry and Molecular Biology (T.S. Work and E. Work, eds), p. 399. Elsevier, Amsterdam.
10. Kohn, H. (1970) J. Clin. Pathol. 23, 733.
11. Laurell, C.-B. (1966) Anal. Biochem. 15, 45.
12. Laurell, C.-B. and McKay, E.J. (1981) Meth. Immunol. 73, 339.
13. Ganrot, P.O. (1972) Scand. J. Clin. Lab. Invest. 29, (Suppl.) 124, 39.
14. Axelsen, N.H. (ed.) (1983) Handbook of Immunoprecipitaton-in-Gel Techniques. Blackwell Scientific Publications, Oxford.
15. Gaechtgens, W. (1906) Munchen med. Wchnschr. 53, 135.
16. Boyden, S.V. (1951) J. Exp. Med. 93, 107.
17. Leuvering, J.W.H. et al. (1980) J. Immunoassay 1, 77.
18. Cais, M. (1983) Meth. Enzymol. 92, 445.
19. Singer, J.M. and Plotz, C.M. (1956) Am. J. Med. 21, 888.
20. Levinski, R.J. and Soothill, J.F. (1977) Clin Exp. Immunol. 29, 428.
21. Grange, J. et al. (1977) J. Immunol. Methods 18, 365.

43. von Schulthess, G.K. et al. (1976) Immunochemistry 13, 963.

Chapter 10

1. Ekins, R.P. (1992) in Developments of Radioimmunoassay and Related Procedures–Proceedings Symposium, Vienna 1991, p. 3. International Atomic Energy Agency, Vienna.
2. Green, M. et al. (1991) in Principles and Practice of Immunoassay (C.P. Price and D.J. Newman, eds), p. 482. Macmillan, London and Stockton Press, New York.
3. Sutherland, R. et al. (1991) in Principles and Practice of Immunoassays (C.P. Price and D.J. Newman, eds), p. 515. Macmillan, London and Stockton Press, New York.
4. Malan, P.G. (1994) in The Immunoassay Handbook (D. Wild, ed.), p. 125. Macmillan, London and Stockton Press, New York.

Chapter 11

1. Rodbard, D. et al. (1969) J. Lab. Clin. Med. 74/5, 770.
2. Finney, D.J. (1983) Clin. Chem. 29/10, 1762.
3. Vogt, W. et al. (1987) Clin. Chim. Acta. 87, 101.
4. Raab, G.M. (1981) Appl. Stat. 30, 32.
5. Rodbard, D. (1974) Clin. Chem. 20, 1255.

6. Ekins, R.P. and Newman, B. (1970) *Acta Endocrinol.* (Suppl) **147**, 11.
7. Malan, P.G. *et al.* (1978) in *Radioimmunoassay and Related Procedures in Medicine*, p. 425. International Atomic Energy Agency, Vienna.
8. Wilkins, T.A. *et al.* (1978) in *Radioimmunoassay and Related Procedures in Medicine*, p. 399. International Atomic Energy Agency, Vienna.
9. Hawker, F.J. and Challand, G.S. (1981) *Clin. Chem.* **27**, 14.
10. Ekins, R.P. (1983) *Immunoassays for Clinical Chemistry*, p. 76. Churchill Livingstone, Edinburgh.
11. Rodbard, D. (1978) *Anal. Biochem.* **90**, 1.
12. Shewhart, W.A. (1931) *Economic Control of Quality of the Manufactured Product*. van Nostrand, NY.
13. Kemp, K.W. *et al.* (1978) *J. Endocrinol.* **76**, 203.
14. Westgard, J.O. *et al.* (1981) *Clin. Chem.* **27**, 493.
15. Raab, G.M. *et al.* (1985) *Clin. Chem.* **31**, 1264.

INDEX

ESSENTIAL DATA SERIES

All researchers need rapid access to data on a daily basis. The *Essential Data* series provides this core information in convenient pocket-sized books. For each title, the data have been carefully chosen, checked and organized by an expert in the subject area. *Essential Data* books therefore provide the information that researchers need in the form in which they need it.

Centrifugation. *D. Rickwood, T.C. Ford & J. Steensgaard*
0 471 94271 5, 1994, £12.99/$19.95

Gel Electrophoresis. *D. Patel*
0 471 94306 1, 1994, £12.99/$19.95

Light Microscopy. *C. Rubbi*
0 471 94270 7, 1994, £12.99/$19.95

Vectors. *P. Gacesa & D. Ramji*
0 471 94841 1, 1994, £12.99/$19.95

Human Cytogenetics. *D. Rooney & B. Czepulkowski (Eds)*
0 471 95076 9, 1994, £12.99/$19.95

Animal Cells: culture and media. *D.C. Darling & S.J. Morgan*
0 471 94300 2, 1994, £12.99/$19.95

Cell and Molecular Biology. *D. Rickwood & D. Patel*
0 471 95568 X, 1995, £14.99/$23.95

PCR. *C.R. Newton (Ed.)*
0 471 95222 2, 1995, £14.99/$23.95

Nucleic Acid Hybridization. *P.M. Gilmartin*
0 471 95084 X, 1996, £12.99/$19.95

Immunoassays. *R. Edwards (Ed.)*
0 471 95275 3, 1996, £12.99/$19.95

ORDER FORM

Please send me:

Qty	Title	Price/copy	Total
.....	....	....	....
.....	....	....	....
.....	....	....	....
.....	....	....	....

All prices correct at time of going to press but subject to change. Your order will be processed without delay, please allow 21 days for delivery. We will refund your payment without question if you return any unwanted book to us in resaleable condition within 30 days. All books are available from your bookseller.

Method of payment

☐ Payment £/$ _____ enclosed (payable to John Wiley & Sons Ltd). Orders for one book only – please add £3.00/$4.95 to cover postage and handling. Two or more books postage FREE.

☐ Purchase order enclosed

☐ Please send me an invoice (£3.00/$4.95 will be added to cover postage and handling)

☐ Please charge my credit card account
  ☐ American Express ☐ Diners Club
  ☐ Visa ☐ Mastercard

Card no. |_____| Expiry: |_____|

Signature: _____

Telephone our Customer Services Dept with your cash or credit card order on 01243 829121 or dial FREE on 0800 243407 (UK only)

Send my order to:

Name (PLEASE PRINT) _____

Position: _____

Address: _____

_____

_____

Telephone: _____

Signature: _____ Date: _____

Return to: Rebecca Harfield, John Wiley & Sons Ltd, Baffins Lane, Chichester, West Sussex PO19 1UD, UK. Telefax: (01243) 775878

or: Wiley-Liss, 605 Third Avenue, New York, NY 10158-0012, USA. Telefax: (212) 850-8888

☐ If you do not wish to receive mailings from other companies please tick this box or notify the Marketing Services Department at John Wiley & Sons Ltd.

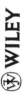 WILEY

Printed and bound by CPI Group (UK) Ltd, Croydon, CR0 4YY

16/04/2025

14658502-0001